Clinical Guidelines and The Law

Negligence, Discretion and Judgment

Brian Hurwitz

General Practitioner, London and
Senior Lecturer in General Practice
Imperial College School of Medicine

Foreword by

Sir Douglas Black

Radcliffe Medical Press

© 1998 Brian Hurwitz

Radcliffe Medical Press Ltd
18 Marcham Road, Abingdon, Oxon OX14 1AA, UK

British Library Cataloguing in Publication Data

A catalogue record for this book is available from the British Library.

ISBN 1 85775 044 6

Library of Congress Cataloging-in-Publication Data is available.

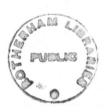

Typesest by Acorn Bookwork, Salisbury, Wilts.
Printed and bound by Redwood Books, Trowbridge, Wilts.

Contents

Foreword

There are nine and sixty ways of constructing tribal lays,
And – every – single – one – of – them – is – right.

Kipling can scarcely have had medical guidelines in mind when he
wrote these words but the first of his lines could be applied to them, in
their infinite variety; the second line, emphatically, could not. Aphor-
istic codifications of medical experience are arresting but they are also
distorting. Just as sound-bites are no substitute for reasoned argument,
guidelines cannot encompass the rich variety and built-in impermanence
of currently accepted medical knowledge, and still less the subtleties of
its application to the care of individual patients. These few sentences
express a vague unease which I have long felt about the proliferation of
algorithms, pseudo-categorical imperatives and directives by which the
practice of medicine is now surrounded.

Brian Hurwitz has now supplied an extended critical analysis of the
different types of formulation which come under the general heading of
'guidelines' and goes on to consider the degree of authority which
different guidelines may carry, and the manner in which they may be
used. His chapter on the nature and context of clinical guidance illus
trates copiously the many guises in which it may come and the range of
its sources, from statutory authorities through universities and medical
Colleges to individual authors. This diversity of origin has a bearing on
the authority of particular elements of clinical advice: some guidelines
specify procedures which are enjoined or else prohibited by statute,
while others do no more than indicate a generally acceptable course of
practice. Even governmental guidelines are not necessarily clear-cut, as
is well shown in a reply given by Lady Thatcher in the course of the
Scott Enquiry. In reply to a question on whether guidelines are expected
to be followed, she said, 'Of course they have to be followed. They
need to be followed for what they are, guidelines.'

Guidance flows in such quantity and in such varied forms – codes,
directives, circulars and administrative letters – from the NHS authorities that there may be a problem in teasing out from it what are truly
'guidelines'. One suggested definition, from the Institute of Medicine in
the USA, gives 'systematically developed statements to assist practitioner
and patient decisions about appropriate health care for specific clinical

circumstances', a formulation in which the word *'assist'* deserves and even demands particular emphasis. The exercise of distilling summary statements from the natural history of disease, including the effects of its treatment, is certainly educational for the author, as anyone knows who has tried to do it or even written a textbook article. If the task is performed well, it can truly educate the reader and assist the practitioner.

The benefits of well-constructed guidelines have to be weighed against the hazards of ill-constructed guidelines which confer a spurious authority on a statement (perhaps even a memorable one) which is the result of an incomplete or even flawed analysis. But that is not the most serious danger of 'rule-book medicine', based on guidelines of variable quality. That danger is seen by Dr Hurwitz as its possible effects on 'the way doctors practise and the manner in which they are to be held accountable'. He finds that the difference between 'skills grounded in practical experience' and 'those based merely on following instruction or obeying rules' was recognized as far back as Plato; but he suggests that nowadays 'the climate and framework in which health care is provided increasingly emphasizes the value of standardized treatments promoted by guidelines'.

There is perhaps no present danger that the standard of 'accepted professional skills and methods', will be replaced by 'adherence to official guidelines'; but at some distant date the Pharisee and the reductionist might discover and explore dangerous common ground in a system of medical accountability based on a rule book, itself a compote of guidelines. As this book shows, the treatment of illness cannot be comprehended within a formulation analogous to the 'trouble-shooting' section in a manual such as may accompany a washing-machine or video recorder.

Douglas Black
March 1998

Acknowledgements

I have two major intellectual debts in writing this book – to Professors Ian Kennedy and Andrew Grubb of the Centre for Medical Law and Ethics, King's College, London, who first kindled my interest in medical law and negligence, and to the Clinical Guidelines Group of the Royal College of General Practitioners of which I was a member: Professors Allen Hutchinson and Martin Eccles, and Drs Jeremy Grimshaw, Gene Feder, Richard Baker and Martin Lawrence with all of whom I had many lively discussions during 1993/94.

I would particularly like to thank Jeremy Grimshaw for allowing me access to the extensive bibliography of clinical guidelines which he has built up in the Department of Health Services Research, University of Aberdeen; Robin Downie, Professor of Moral Philosophy at Glasgow University who made helpful comments on an early draft of two chapters; and Dr Phil Cotton, of the Department of General Practice at Glasgow who kept an eye out for useful references.

I would also like to thank the staff of the libraries at the Institute of Advanced Legal Studies, University of London, and at the British Medical Association, for help in locating relevant materials.

I thank my dear wife, Dr Ruth Richardson, without whose support the book might not have been started and without whose encouragement it would not yet have been completed; and my dear mother who cared for our son during the process of proofreading. Needless to say, I alone am responsible for any misinterpretations or errors.

For dear Ruth and Joshua

Introduction

This book is designed to address the cultural and philosophical unease frequently felt by potential users and developers of clinical guidelines about the increasingly important place guidelines are now accorded in health care systems. Knowing exactly what makes a guideline a guideline and whether guidelines carry greater authority than other clinical advisory statements, such as textbooks, is fundamental to creating a cultural framework in which health care professionals can fluently use (or reject) guidelines. But even more important than this is a full discussion of the kind of liability to which guideline users, authors and sponsors may be exposed. The book explores these professional and legal issues, and focuses upon conceptual tensions that have arisen between differing notions of clinical guidelines.

Statements of clinical guidance purporting to be 'guidelines' have become a commonplace of UK medical practice. Articles published in medical journals are now ten times more likely to refer to 'guidelines' than 25 years ago.[1] But although guideline effectiveness studies are a new focus of research, how often doctors consult them, and to what effect, remains unknown.[2,3]

The development and sponsorship of clinical guidelines in the UK is currently undertaken by a wide variety of organizations, including the Department of Health, medical and surgical Royal Colleges, specialist associations, purchasing authorities, hospital providers, general practitioners, patient organizations and private medical providers. Guideline use, it is hoped, will offer patients a guarantee of effective, consistent, and up-to-date treatment. Proclaimed by their advocates as powerful instruments of assistance to clinicians, capable of extending the clinical roles of nurses and pharmacists, and seen by purchasers and managers as technological tools guaranteeing treatment quality, guidelines *also* offer mechanisms by which doctors and other health care professionals can be made more accountable for their clinical activities.[3]

Despite this remarkable ascendancy within medicine, clinical guidelines make up, as yet, only a small part of an expanding web of rules, recommendations and advisory statements by which society seeks to regulate many diverse activities. In public affairs, guidelines are held to govern the conduct of cabinet ministers, the sale of arms to foreign countries, the operation of professional parliamentary lobby groups, and even the sexual probity of Church of England clergy.[4] Applications for memberships and mortgages, for grants or free gifts, are equally likely to be accompanied with requests to follow *guidelines*, designed (it appears), to ensure that such applications are made 'in a proper manner'. Hence guidelines feature on packaged food labels as re-heating and cooking guidelines, and in documentation sent by medical journals to aspiring contributors, such as 'guidelines for authors' and 'guidelines for referees'.[5,6]

Authority, it has been claimed, is indissoluably connected with the notion of a rule-governed form of life, to the notion that there are correct and incorrect ways of doing things which can be specified by rules.[7] A dialogue which took place during the Scott Inquiry into the Arms for Iraq Affair illustrates the appeal guidelines hold to those attempting to enforce accountability upon professionals who have traditionally regarded their work as self-directed, and generally free from outside interference.[8]

'Ms Baxendale QC: Some of the witnesses we have had have described these guidelines as a framework, within which to work ... Does that fit in with how you saw the guidelines?

Lady Thatcher: They are exactly what they say, guidelines, they are not the law. They are guidelines.

Ms Baxendale QC: Did they have to be followed?

Lady Thatcher: Of course they have to be followed, but they are not strict law. That is why they are guidelines and not law and, of course, they have to be applied according to the relevant circumstances.

Ms Baxendale QC: They are expected to be followed?

Lady Thatcher: Of course they have to be followed. They need to be followed for what they are, guidelines.'[9]

Issues raised in this exchange are also at the heart of concerns addressed by this book: whether guidelines carry appropriate authority, and in which circumstances they should properly be viewed as imposing mandatory obligations upon doctors.

The National Health Service Executive (NHSE) has observed that clinical guidelines can take the form of 'anything from a set of prescriptive rules (with sanctions for non-compliance), to a voluntary code for self regulation'. It believes the term should be understood as referring to 'a variety of documents produced to meet different needs. Some guidelines have more to do with the agreed protocols of interaction between health service organizations than direct relevance to decisions by clinicians about therapeutic management.'[10]

If health care professionals adopt them, valid clinical guidelines will undoubtedly influence patient care, and pervasive effects could result from their incorporation into the incentive structure of the health service.[11] Doctors and health care workers should therefore be knowledgeable about guideline literature so that they can readily identify and reject bizarre or invalid protocols or guidelines which emanate from factional interests.[12]

I believe that valid clinical guidelines can assist doctors in providing appropriate and up-to-date medical care to patients in many clinical situations, but that insufficient attention has been paid by the developers and issuers of guidelines, to the clinical complexities and uncertainties of every day practice. How guideline and user are intended to interact and what model of clinical judgment is embedded in a guideline, are rarely made explicit. By stimulating open debate about these issues, it is hoped this book will contribute to the newly emerging professional disciplines of clinical guideline development and clinical guideline use.

The position a protocol or guideline occupies in a spectrum starting with permissive advice at one end extending to mandatory commands at the other, may be highly influential in fashioning a purchaser's view of it, and doctors' responses to it. Additional factors may also be important, such as whether incentives are provided for guideline implementation.[13] While UK purchasers are being urged to buy not treatments, but treatment protocols, French doctors have been fined up to £2000 for transgressing any one of 147 clinical guideline statements established with statutory backing.[14–16]

This is all a far cry from 50 years ago, when the autonomy granted to clinicians to practise according to professionally generated standards seemed almost untouched by external regulation. As far back as 1946, alerted by government proposals for a state sponsored health service, a British Medical Association committee announced that in any future health service:

'The medical profession should remain free to exercise the art and science of medicine according to its traditions, standards and knowledge, the individual doctor retaining full responsibility for the care of the patient, freedom of judgment... without interference in his professional work.'[17]

Clinical freedom on such a scale has been progressively curtailed in the UK in the past 20 years, and this has coincided with an explosion of guideline statements. But are guidelines the cause of this curtailment, or a symptom of it? Guideline proliferation has not been confined to countries with state funded health services. In the USA, some 20 000 health care standards and clinical practice guidelines are reported to have been issued by over 500 organizations, including third party payers, peer review organizations, and agencies of – or responsible to – government.[18] American physicians now believe themselves to be 'pinioned by regulations and controls far beyond... colleagues in most other countries'.[19]

But what exactly are clinical guidelines? Should they be viewed as technological embodiments of medical knowledge that require evaluation like any other piece of new medical technology? How do they differ from other varieties of clinical guidance, such as standard medical textbooks? Should guidelines be viewed as advisory or mandatory? What sorts of regulatory functions do guidelines serve; have the courts accorded guidelines any credence, and do guidelines allow sufficient room for clinical discretion? This book addresses these questions, and aims to provide readers with sufficient knowledge of the literature to contribute to the growing debate about the role of clinical guidelines in modern health care.[12]

Chapter 1 critically examines various definitions of clinical guidelines, relating them to current usage and to a cluster of technical terms such as 'protocol' and 'review criterion'. Chapter 2 distinguishes and dissects the notions of guideline authority and guideline validity and discusses their critical appraisal. Many of the issues which the book addresses are not new – as we shall see in a moment. In the 3rd century BC, Plato discussed the significance of what would happen if doctors' activities were to become bound by clinical rules-of-thumb not dissimilar from the modern notion of guidelines. However, what *is* new is the growing realization, now acknowledged by the NHSE, that clinical guidelines can play a role in legal disputes.[20] Despite concerns about their variable quality, the Government wants to see more and more clinical guidelines developed and used across the NHS as a means of promoting best practice, and proposes to create a National Institute of Clinical Excellence to take the lead in developing and disseminating cost-effective guidelines.[21] This book offers readers a comprehensive guide to the medico-legal issues likely to arise from this development.

Do doctors who deviate from guidelines place themselves at increased risk of being found liable if patients suffer injury as a result? Could compliance with guidelines protect health care workers from liability in such circumstances? What legal responsibility do the developers and issuers of guidelines have if their guidance is found to be faulty? These questions are addressed in detail in Chapters 3, 4 and 5, and readers who already have a good grasp of the general issues raised by guidelines may wish to turn immediately to these chapters.

Chapter 3 outlines how clinical guidelines have come to feature in the legal arena, focusing upon examples of UK, European, and US legislation that use guidelines as regulatory devices. Chapter 4 introduces the concept of negligence, and discusses common law cases featuring clinical guidelines or protocols, and explains how the courts go about determining the legal status of such guidance. Cases from UK, US and Commonwealth jurisdictions are mentioned, and further information on each case is provided in Appendix 1.

Chapter 5 explores the challenges that evidence-based practice and evidence-linked guidelines may pose to the traditional standard of medical care expected by the courts, examines legal issues of guideline author liability, and addresses the importance which the courts can attach to clinical discretion.[22] A discussion of the nature of guideline use, and its interaction with clinical judgment and clinical freedom is to be found in Chapter 6. An annotated bibliography of key cases cited appears in Appendix 1, and a selected annotated further reading list in Appendix 2.

References

1 Medline computer search by the author for the years 1973–93.
2 Grimshaw JM and Russell IT (1993) The effect of clinical guidelines on medical practice: a systematic review of rigorous evaluations. *Lancet.* **2**: 1317–22.
3 NHS Centre for Reviews and Dissemination (1994) Implementing clinical practice guidelines. *Effective Health Care Bulletin.* **8**; Clinical Guidelines Working Group (1995) Preface. In: *The Development and Implementation of Clinical Guidelines. Report from General Practice Number 26.* RCGP, London.
4 Bosely S (1996) Guide lists ways to help clergy keep sexual pitfalls at bay. *The Guardian.* **24 Sept**: 6.
5 Anonymous (1991) Guidelines for writing papers. *BMJ.* **302**: 40.
6 Anonymous (1991) Guidelines for referees. *BMJ.* **302**: 41.
7 Peters RS (1996) *Ethics and Education.* Allen and Unwin, London, pp. 237–65.

8 Scott R (1996) *Report of the Inquiry into the Export of Defence Equipment and Dual-Use Goods to Iraq and Related Prosecutions.* HMSO, London. This report, which took three years to compile, ran to over a million words in its consideration of whether four guidelines, expressed in a mere 80 words, concerning the sale of arms to Iran and Iraq, had or had not been breached. The guidelines were originally drawn up by officials from the Foreign Office and the Ministry of Defence, and also concerned the Department of Trade and Industry. Each government department apparently had its own view about the degree of flexibility permitted by the guidelines.

9 Norton-Taylor R (1995) Half the Picture. In: Norton-Taylor R and Lloyd M (eds) *Truth is a Difficult Concept: inside the Scott Inquiry.* A Guardian Book, Fourth Estate Ltd, London, pp. 213–74.

10 NHS Executive (1996) *Clinical Guidelines: using clinical guidelines to improve patient care within the NHS.* DoH, London, p. 9.

11 NHS Management Executive (1993) and (1994) *Improving Clinical Effectiveness.* Department of Health, Leeds. EL(93)115 and EL(94)74.

12 Royal College of General Practitioners (1995) Guideline effectiveness – the pitfalls and obstacles. In: *The Development and Implementation of Clinical Guidelines. Report from General Practice Number 26.* RCGP, London, pp. 3–7.

13 Department of Health (1993) *The National Health Service Statement of Fees and Allowances.* Para. 30 Sch. 1–5. DoH, Welsh Office, London.

14 Williams A (1994) How should information on cost-effectiveness influence clinical practice? In: Delamothe T (ed.) *Outcomes into Clinical Practice.* BMJ Publishing Group, London, p. 100.

15 Durand-Zaleski I, Colin C and Blum-Boisgard C (1997) An attempt to save money using mandatory practice guidelines in France. *BMJ.* 315: 943–6.

16 Dixon J (1997) France seeks to curb health costs by fining doctors. *BMJ.* 315: 895–6.

17 British Medical Association (1946) *Negotiating Committee Report.* BMA, London.

18 Leone A (1993) Medical practice guidelines are useful tools in litigation. *Medical Malpractice: Law & Strategy.* 10: 1–6.

19 Silver G (1987) Discordant priorities. *Lancet.* i: 1195.

20 NHS Executive (1996) *Clinical Guidelines. Using Clinical Guidelines to Improve Patient Care within the NHS.* DoH, London, p. 10.

21 Secretary of State for Health (1997) *The New NHS* (Cmnd 3807). HMSO, London.

22 National Health and Medical Research Council (1995) Legal impli-
    cations of guidelines. In: *Guidelines for the Development and
    Implementation of Clinical Guidelines*. Australian Government
    Publishing Service, Canberra, pp. 27–8.

1 The Nature and Context of Clinical Guidance

Over 5000 statements are issued annually by the National Health Service Executive (NHSE) and other health service agencies consisting of guidance, executive letters and official instructions.[1] An expert in health law has observed that 'these circulars and other such literature are not "law" in the sense in which lawyers would use the term. Nevertheless they are highly important guides to conduct...'[2] and can be influential upon the outcome of a court's deliberations, such as in judicial review of local health policies.[3]

Many of these statements refer to financial and administrative matters, but a significant number concern clinical policy and service guidance which the NHSE has recognized 'may incorporate components of clinical guidelines'.[4] Letters from the Chief Medical and Nursing Officers, publications such as *Prescribers' Journal*, *Health Trends* and those of the Medicines Resource Centre are concerned explicitly with clinical guidance, and are distributed free of charge to practising doctors as a matter of public health policy.

A Department of Health sponsored report identified the confused status of many of these statements: 'GPs and practice managers find it difficult to discern what is for action, what is for guidance and what is merely for reference'.[5]

Should clinical advisory statements be issued only if accompanied by one of three possible labels; 'for action', denoting that it be obeyed as instructed; 'for guidance' implying advice to be heeded with appropriate discretion; 'for reference' meaning for consultation only? Where do clinical guidelines fit into this classification?

Guideline definitions

In the introduction to a widely read textbook of medicine, the physician and teacher, Maurice Pappworth, cautioned students to look critically at the invention of new terms because they may disguise failures of understanding. He cited Goethe's observation that 'when true concept fails us, an idle word steps in to take its place'.[6]

Through overusage and misapplication, 'guideline' risks attaining just such an 'idle' status. Partridge's *Usage and Abusage* classes it amongst 'vogue words', a group of 'lowly humdrum words raised to high estate' which thereby acquire a power and an influence beyond their desert.[7]

For a term that has found application in areas as diverse as cooking, cabinet conduct and clinical medicine, we should not be surprised to discover that 'guideline' lacks a distinctive definition. According to the *Oxford English Dictionary* a 'guideline' can be an aid to manual activity, as used in the phrase 'guideline for a saw'. The American *Random House Dictionary of the English Language* elaborates a metaphorical usage, defining 'guideline' as 'a rope or cord that serves to guide one's steps', or 'a guide or indication of a future course of action'. 'To guide', in this context, means 'to supply with advice or counsel', indicating 'continuous presence or agency in showing or indicating a course'.[8] Hence a guideline may be compared with its more pictorial counterpart, a blueprint, in defining both a plan of action and the course by which the plan will unfold and be realized.

In clinical medicine, 'guideline' is frequently to be found in the company of a cluster of other technical terms seeking to define and to patrol the shifting boundaries between acceptable (effective) practice, and poor (ineffective) practice. The meanings of these terms are not always easily distinguished from each other.

Protocol

Protocol is a term referring originally to the first page of a manuscript, or a formal proceeding duly attested, and now shares with 'guideline' the generic aim of providing guidance to practising doctors. The general purpose of clinical protocols is to direct clinicians along preferred treatment pathways by outlining detailed management plans for discrete clinical conditions judged amenable to step-wise decision-making processes specifiable in flow diagrams, or algorithms.[9,10] Protocols tend to be viewed as more restrictive than guidelines, making their relevance in clinical settings questionable. According to one influential opinion:

'protocols that attempt to define what should happen to a patient with a particular condition are dangerous territory, drawing on fears of inflexibility and the dangers of defensive medicine. Altogether a protocol seems too firm for the uncertain business of clinical practice. A guideline at least leaves some latitude.'[11]

The Scottish Clinical Resource and Audit Group has attempted to reserve the term 'protocol' for the detailed *local* development (at practice, hospital or unit level) of nationally agreed guidelines.[12] However, this particular meaning of 'protocol' is not yet widely accepted outside Scotland.

Practice policies

Practice policies consist of agreed courses of action in particular clinical areas. Practice policies 'identify the available options, estimate the consequences of different options, and determine the desirability of those outcomes to patients'. They can be thought of as generic decisions which direct clinical practices in certain directions rather than others for collections of patients or for a single patient.[13]

Medical review criteria

Medical review criteria are designed to allow assessment of health care quality, the appropriateness of clinical decisions, services or outcomes.[8] Review criteria can be constructed from guidelines by specifying discrete measurable aspects of clinical activity that accurately assess compliance with a guideline. An example from the British Hypertension Society Guidelines has been suggested; these state that 'great emphasis should be placed on encouraging patients to stop smoking...' from which the following review criteria have been constructed. Medical records should show that at least annually:

- there has been assessment of smoking habit, and
- appropriate advice has been given to smokers.

Such criteria, it has been suggested, aim to 'make clear what information is required to assess clinician compliance, how the information is to be obtained, and the time period in which smoking should be assessed'.[14] Notice, however, that in this case such criteria insist upon requirements additional to those in the guideline itself, which makes no mention of record-keeping nor any mention of how frequently advice about smoking should be offered to patients.

Standards of health care quality

Standards of health care quality are frequently formulated as the percentage of processes or events which need to be accomplished by a health care provider. The Institute of Medicine believes they should declare the level of health care quality which they represent, such as:

- a range of acceptable performance or results, or
- minimum levels of acceptable performance or results, or
- excellent levels of performance or results.[8]

For practical purposes, standards of health care quality must be authoritative statements appropriate to particular health care settings. How authority is assessed in the context of clinical guidelines is discussed in the next chapter.

Performance measures

Performance measures are 'methods or instruments to measure the extent to which the actions of health care practitioners conform to practice guidelines, policies, medical review criteria, or standards of quality'.[8]

Codes of practice

Codes of practice refer to sets of recommendations encompassing the safety and efficacy of clinical practices. They may go beyond discrete aims by providing answers to, or frameworks for approaching, 'fundamental ethical and social questions' thrown up by clinical practice.[15] A former Law Lord has emphasized that medical practice requires, as a matter of law, 'that doctors should concern themselves with values and rules outside the limits of clinical judgment'.[16] Whether legally enforceable or not, codes of practice offer mechanisms for facilitating ethically acceptable and socially sensitive practice.

Many of these terms signify notions of health care regulation akin to that of guideline and can, in fact, be viewed as transformed versions of guideline statements fashioned for use by different health care functionaries (such as purchasers, commissioning agencies or regulators) for use in varying health care settings.[17] In the context of this proliferation of technical terms, how are we to understand the difference between guidance and guidelines; and do such statements of recommendation differ from material available from traditional textbooks of medicine?

Guidance, guidelines and textbooks of medicine

Guidelines usually focus upon quite specific issues of clinical management such as the detection, treatment or referral of patients with discrete conditions such as hypertension, asthma, diabetes or infertility. Clinical guidance or guidelines are *not* usually concerned with background questions of aetiology and pathophysiology, matters traditionally well-covered by medical textbooks, but rather with how to optimize treatment decisions in the light of up-to-date and reliable information on safety, efficacy, patient choice, and cost effectiveness.

Textbooks of medicine aim to offer comprehensive assessments of medical conditions divorced from the pressing issues of health services provision. The *Oxford Textbook of Medicine*, for example, states its intention 'to map out the terrain where the physician will face and try to solve the problems of diagnosis and treatment'.[18] Outlining a map is a different process from defining a route. In the case of textbooks, whether a specific treatment should be offered to a particular patient in the singular circumstances of an individual's case is to be left to the appropriately tutored discretion of the clinician in charge of medical care, in the light of all the circumstances. As the *Oxford Textbook of Medicine* states at the outset:

'Textbooks outline the treatment of the diseases described, but physicians do not treat diseases, they treat human beings, all of whom differ from each other, with individual likes and dislikes, fears and prejudices, a unique set of genes, and widely differing environmental backgrounds.'[18]

Guidelines, by comparison, are more concerned with specifying treatment strategies for certain patient types, with health care quality, and the reduction of unjustifiable clinical variability and costs. Guidelines tend to focus upon measurable outcomes of health care in the light of actual limited health resources available to a locality, or within a particular sector of the NHS. In offering pre-fabricated treatment strategies, guidelines tend to be more *directive* of clinicians, adopting the phraseology of the moral imperative, than do traditional textbooks of medicine.

Another way of looking at a guideline is as a collection of recommendations embodying certain standards of clinical management. By analogy with a plumbline which is governed by a physical principle, gravity, and which authoritatively delineates a standard (the vertical), a clinical guideline can be viewed as staking out a standard of practice. But unlike a plumbline – which is governed by a reliable and invariable force – clinical guidelines are not transparent indicators of the workings and fabric of the natural world, but the products of complex development strategies which may more or less adequately match agreed standards. Elaborated by processes which can seem a far cry from clinical practice, guidelines could propose standards of care that meet, fall below, or are superior to customary standards of clinical practice.[19,20]

Despite their variable quality (further discussed in the next chapter), clinical guidelines are established components of the cultural and economic changes which are taking place in health services provision. Their proliferation to some extent reflects the changing regulatory framework of health care in the UK which is changing from one in which professional stewardship of medical provision once predominated, towards a framework dominated by civil regulation and quasi-market mechanisms. The broad legal effects of these changes have been eloquently outlined by Ian Kennedy, a distinguished expert on medical law:

'The sense of belonging to a flawed but noble enterprise where everyone gained a little bit, where the system tried to do its best for all by all, is going. The language is now of consumers, providers, purchasers, charters, enterprise, targets. These changes in ethos will produce a sea change in the role of recourse to law. The law deals every day with the language of consumers, users, charters, purchasers and contracts. This is the language of law, especially when coupled with accompanying rhetoric about rights.'[21]

Under the new regime Professor Kennedy predicts that 'the role of protocols and guidelines will become more and more significant in determining whether a doctor has violated the law'.[21] The reasons for this are complex and are discussed in depth in Chapter 5, but to the extent that clinical guidelines successfully encapsulate consensus standards of medical care, departure from such guidelines may be viewed by the courts as requiring special justification if patients suffer harm as a result.

Currently, clinical guidelines originate from many organizations of differing authority, and can embody widely variable aims and values. For this reason, the NHSE has outlined its strategy for commending clinical guidelines to the NHS, including the prioritization and evidence-based criteria which it wishes to see adopted for guideline selection.[22] Only guidelines based upon randomized controlled trials, and/or expert opinion (endorsed by 'respected authorities') will be considered eligible for commendation.

The NHSE sees a valuable role for guidelines in the following circumstances:

- where there is excessive morbidity, disability or mortality
- where treatment offers good potential for reducing morbidity, disability or mortality
- where there is wide variation in clinical practice
- where the services involved are resource intensive
- where medical care of a condition involves 'many boundary issues' cutting across primary, secondary and community care and across professional boundaries.[22]

Approved guidelines currently represent a small fraction of the total number of clinical guidelines in circulation. Health care professionals therefore need to be in a position to evaluate the validity and applicability of clinical guidelines, as well as their possible legal significance. This task is made difficult by the sheer ubiquity of guidelines, and is compounded by the tendency for terms such as 'policy', 'recommendation', 'protocol', and 'guideline' to be used loosely, even interchangeably, in a medical context. An instructive example of such interchangeability at work is revealed by the Gillick case. In 1981, Victoria Gillick wrote to her local Area Health Authority expressing concern about 'new DHSS Guidelines on the contraceptive and abortion treatment of children under both the legal and medical age of consent'.[23] Although the DHSS circular that sparked her letter had not used the term 'guideline', the reply which she received from the chairman of her Area Health Authority adopted Mrs Gillick's term, and offered a particular gloss on the relationship between guidelines and clinical discretion:

'We would expect our doctors to work within these guidelines but, as the Minister has stated, the final decision in these matters must be one of clinical judgment.'[24]

Believing this advice to be both morally flawed and unlawful, Mrs Gillick mounted a sustained (but ultimately unsuccessful) public law challenge to the lawfulness of the DHSS circular.[24]

Slippage in linguistic usage of 'guideline' is also manifested by a tendency for the term to supplant medical advisory statements previously designated 'advice', 'recommendation' or 'guidance'. This tendency operates in many contexts: in an article entitled *Guidelines on death certification and referrals to the coroner*, the Royal College of General Practitioners reminds its members that a 1996 letter from the Chief Medical Officer 'updates *guidance* from 1990 on death certification...'.[25] Similarly, the 1994 statement from the Driver and Vehicle Licensing Agency entitled *Fitness to drive: updated guidelines for cardiovascular fitness in vocational drivers*, revises previous advice entitled *Fitness to drive: updated guidance on cardiac conditions in vocational and other professional drivers.*[26,27]

In view of Pappworth's cautions concerning the invention of terminology, we need to question why these statements are appearing in re-labelled forms. What sort of goals are 'guidelines' thought able to achieve which 'guidance' is deemed less likely to achieve? The more recent recommendations, designated guidelines, differ significantly from those they have replaced. The decision to replace 'guidance' with 'guidelines' appears to confer a superadded authority upon the later statements. By invoking the notion of a clinical and moral line that seeks to define the boundary between morally acceptable and less acceptable clinical activity – perhaps even forbidden practices – the term 'guideline' appears to denote more coercive instruction than did its more permissive predecessors.

However, as we have seen, it may not be possible to maintain clear semantic boundaries between guidelines, guidance and recommendations. In an attempt to prevent the meaning of guideline becoming stretched 'to include too many different kinds of guidance',[28] the US Institute of Medicine, which until recently had a statutory responsibility to commission clinical guidelines, developed a definition of guideline which has been widely adopted. In its view, guidelines should be viewed as:

'systematically developed statements to assist practitioner and patient decisions about appropriate health care for specific clinical circumstances.'[29]

This formulation has gained acceptance in the UK as an encapsulation of the essential elements that clinical guidance should attain in order to be granted the upgraded designation of guidelines.[30] Formal and systematic methods of development are required to ensure that guideline recommendations are as evidence-based as possible. In addition, the scope of a guideline's application requires to be limited to 'specific clinical circumstances' to enable potential users to gain a clear view of the particular situations in which guidelines might be helpful.

The Institute of Medicine's definition, though widely quoted, does not really provide sufficient information to distinguish clinical guidelines from other statements of guidance and recommendation. Nor does it help us to understand why, for example, different systematically developed guidelines, covering the same treatment areas, may yet significantly differ in recommended strategies and treatment thresholds.[31] Differences in the clinical recommendations which expert panels of differing nationality derive from the same research evidence have been documented. Fahey and Peters note that five clinical guidelines on hypertension have been developed systematically using an evidence linked approach, but agree on the diagnosis of 'controlled' hypertension in only 18% of patients, and on 'uncontrolled' hypertension in 13% of cases. Moreover, the proportion of patients classified as controlled varies more than four-fold between these guidelines.[32] The authors note that the same sources of evidence were used in the development of the guidelines, and that:

'All of them used an explicit process to identify and select evidence; what is not clear is how similar studies were combined to produce differing recommendations... The content of national guidelines seems to be influenced by factors other than results from randomised controlled trials. National culture and expectations influence the way in which medical care is organised and delivered, and the variation in content of hypertension guidelines may be a manifestation of the cultural expectations of apparent benefits and risks when treating this condition.'[32]

The same problem has emerged in other clinical areas.[33,34] In deriving recommendations for coronary angiography and coronary bypass from the same scientific studies US experts tend to be more action orientated and interventionist than those from the UK.[35]

The US Evidence-Based Medicine Working Group has tried to define more closely the nature of clinical guidelines. According to its definition, guidelines:

'Like overviews, ... gather, appraise and combine evidence. Guidelines, however, go beyond most overviews in attempting to address all the issues relevant to a clinical decision and all the values that might sway a clinical recommendation. Like decision analysis, guidelines refine clinical questions and balance trade-offs. Guidelines differ from decision analysis in relying more on qualitative reasoning and in emphasising a particular clinical context.'

Guidelines make explicit recommendations, often on behalf of health organizations, with a definite intent to influence what clinicians do. These suggestions about what should be done go beyond a simple presentation of evidence, costs, or decision models. They reflect value judgments about the relative importance of various health and economic outcomes in specific clinical situations. As a result, they should be required to pass unique tests about how matters of opinion, in addition to matters of science, are handled.[36]

This fuller statement is helpful because it hints at the intellectual processes involved in guideline creation, evokes the regulatory effect of guidelines upon medical practice, and acknowledges the role that human values play in the social organization of health care and in the construction and operation of guidelines. The Evidence-Based Medicine Working Group has emphasized that:

'The clinical problems for which practice guidelines are most needed often involve complex trade-offs between competing benefits, harms and costs, usually under conditions of uncertainty. Even in the presence of strong *evidence* from randomised clinical trials, the effect size of an intervention may be marginal or the intervention may be associated with costs, discomforts, or impracticalities that lead to disagreement or ambivalence among guideline developers about what to *recommend*.'[36]

The Director of the UK Cochrane Centre has remarked that it can be easier to agree on which evidence is relevant to a health care question, and what the evidence shows, than it can be to agree on *how* to derive clinical recommendations from such evidence for incorporation into guidelines. Speaking to the 1995 House of Lords Select Committee on Science and Technology Dr Chalmers said:

'Well, the evidence says this. What the implications of the evidence are for practice requires a judgment... one has to distinguish between what the evidence says and what the evidence means.'[37]

Jonathan Lomas, Professor of Health Services Research at McMaster University, argues that guidelines amount to rules which aim to 'establish, control, or change the behaviour of institutions, individuals, or both...', a view that has been reiterated by the NHSE.[4,38] Questions such as who issues the guidelines, and to whom the authors are responsible therefore loom large. Once guidelines are understood in this light, attempts to delineate effective dissemination and implementation approaches to guideline use require to be viewed as attempts to devise strategies to control clinical activities.

Some studies indicate that guideline dissemination is particularly effective if combined with educational initiatives; implementation may be made more effective if combined with reminder prompts.[39] Yet despite these reports, guidelines alone are rarely found to be influential factors in changing the clinical practices of doctors.[40,41] They may be much less potent agents of change than the health care beliefs and practices of local opinion leaders, or the offering of incentives and the removal of disincentives.[42,43] Attempts to increase guideline potency in this respect have led to US claims that legal vulnerability can be decreased by complying with guidelines, though the evidence for this is slim.[44,45] Such approaches may also be making their appearance in the UK. Referring to poor compliance with guidelines recommending annual retinal screening of patients with diabetes, a consultant physician recently announced that 'more litigation with larger damages may be the only way to make purchasers and providers do their job'.[45] Whether such approaches to guideline implementation will increase compliance remains doubtful, but such threats inevitably associate guidelines with a command and control mentality.[47]

In the UK, the courts have taken note of clinical guidelines and, on occasion, have been asked to examine their legal status or required to scrutinize their recommendations. The next chapter examines the authority and standing of guidelines, while Chapters 3, 4 and 5 discuss how guidelines find their way into court proceedings and the roles they can play in assisting courts in their deliberations.

Summary

The term 'guideline' is of modern coinage and there is no single definitive encapsulation of the notion.

In seeking to define (and to patrol) the shifting boundary between morally acceptable and morally less acceptable clinical practice, clinical guidelines vary in their quality, and in the standards of health care which they seek to establish.

References

1   Kerr D (1995) Information implosion. *J Roy Coll Phys Lond*. 29: 265.

2   Finch JD (1981) *Health Services Law*. Sweet & Maxwell, London, p. 29.

3   See for example, R v North Derbyshire Health Authority, *ex parte* Fisher (*Times*. 2 December 1997) which concerned a request by a sufferer of multiple sclerosis, Kenneth Fisher, to be supplied with beta interferon which had been prescribed by his doctor. His local health authority had adopted a policy of not supplying this expen-

sive medication except to patients participating in a national study of the drug's efficacy. This policy was found by Mr Justice Dyson to be unlawful, because it took no account of an NHSE Circular, EL(95)97, which had requested health authorities and providers to manage use of expensive drugs such as beta interferon via hospital prescribing policies and guidelines. Although the Circular had been advisory and not mandatory in both 'substance and form' the judge found that this 'was not a case of a health authority considering national policy and departing from it. The authority was opposed to the policy and decided to disregard it. This was something it was not entitled to do.'

4 NHS Executive (1996) *Clinical Guidelines: using clinical guidelines to improve patient care within the NHS*. DoH, London, p. 10.

5 NHS Executive (1995) *Patients Not Paper*. NHSE, Leeds, p. 47.

6 Pappworth MH (1971) *A Primer of Medicine*. Butterworths, London.

7 Partridge E (1994) *Usage and Abusage: a guide to good English*. (ed. Whitcut J). Hamish Hamilton, London, p. 366.

8 Field M and Lohr K (eds) (1990) *Clinical Practice Guidelines: directions for a new program*. National Academy Press, Washington DC, pp. 8, 37.

9 Schoenbaum S and Gottlieb L (1990) Algorithm based improvement of clinical quality. *BMJ*. **301**: 1374–6.

10 Colman A and Richards B (1993) Clinical algorithms should be standardised. [Letter] *BMJ*. **307**: 443.

11 Hart E (1993) Protocols or guidelines, or neither? *BMJ*. **306**: 816.

12 Clinical Resource and Audit Group (1993) *Clinical Guidelines: a report by a working group set up by the Clinical Resource and Audit Group*. The Scottish Office: National Health Service in Scotland, Edinburgh.

13 Eddy D (1990) Designing a practice policy, standards, guidelines, and options. *JAMA*. **263**: 3077–84.

14 Baker R and Fraser RC (1995) Development of review criteria: linking guidelines and assessment of quality. *BMJ*. **311**: 370–3.

15 Human Fertilisation and Embryology Authority (1991) *Code of Practice*. Document ref. CH(91)5. HFEA, London, p. 1.

16 Lord Scarman (1987) Law and medical practice. In: Byrne P (ed.) *Medicine in Contemporary Society*. King's College and King Edward's Hospital Fund for London, London, pp. 131–9.

17 Kilpatrick R (1994) In the public interest. *Medico-Legal Journal*. **62**/3: 131–47.

18 Cooke AM (1983) On textbooks and medicine. In: Weatherall DJ,

Ledingham JGG and Warrell DA (eds) *Oxford Textbook of Medicine*. Oxford University Press, Oxford, section 1.3–1.5.

19 Feder G (1994) Clinical guidelines in 1994. *BMJ*. **309**: 1457–8.

20 McKee M and Clarke A (1995) Guidelines, enthusiasms, uncertainty, and the limits to purchasing. *BMJ*. **310**: 101–4.

21 Kennedy I (1993) Medicine in society, now and in the future. In: Lock S (ed.) *Eighty-five Not Out: essays to honour Sir George Godber*. King Edward's Hospital Fund for London, London, pp. 69–75.

22 NHS Executive (1996) *Clinical guidelines: using clinical guidelines to improve patient care within the NHS*. DoH, London, pp. 1–30.

23 Kennedy I and Grubb A (1989) *Medical Law: text and materials*. Butterworths, London, pp. 3–4.

24 Gillick v West Norfolk and Wisbech Area Health Authority (1985) 3 *All ER*: 402–37.

25 Anonymous (1996) Guidelines on death certification and referrals to the coroner. *BJGP*. **46**: vii.

26 Irvine J and Petch M (1994) Fitness to drive: updated guidelines for cardiovascular fitness in vocational drivers. *Health Trends*. **26**: 38–40.

27 Gold R and Oliver M (1989) Fitness to drive: updated guidance on cardiac conditions in vocational drivers and other drivers. *Health Trends*. **21**: 88–9.

28 McDonald CJ and Overhage JM (1994) Guidelines you can follow and can trust. *JAMA*. **271**: 872–3.

29 Field M and Lohr K (eds) (1990) *Clinical Practice Guidelines: directions for a new program*. National Academy Press, Washington DC, pp. 8, 14.

30 Royal College of General Practitioners (1995) *The Development and Implementation of Clinical Guidelines*. RCGP, London.

31 Swales JD (1993) Guidelines on guidelines. *J Hypertension*. **11**: 899–903.

32 Fahey TP and Peters TJ (1996) What constitutes controlled hypertension? Patient based comparison of hypertension guidelines. *BMJ*. **313**: 93–6.

33 Clare A (1981) National variations in medical practice. Culture influences medicine more than science does. *BMJ*. **298**: 1334.

34 Hampton JR (1997) Evidence-based medicine, practice variations and clinical freedom. *J Evaluation in Clinical Practice*. **3**: 2, 123–32.

35 Naylor DC (1995) Grey zones of clinical practice: some limits to evidence-based medicine. *Lancet*. **315**: 840–2.

36 Hayward RSA, Wilson MC, Tunis SR *et al.* for the Evidence-Based

Medicine Working Group (1995) Users' guides to the medical literature. *JAMA*. **274**: 570–4.

37 House of Lords' Select Committee on Science and Technology (1995) *Minutes of evidence taken before the Select Committee on Science and Technology*. Sub-committee 1. Medical Research and the NHS Reforms. HL Paper 12–iii:151–67. HMSO, London.

38 Lomas J (1993) Making clinical policy explicit. *Int J Technol Assmt Hlth Care*. **9**: 11–25.

39 Royal College of General Practitioners (1995) Ensuring that guidelines change clinical practice. In: *The Development and Implementation of Clinical Guidelines*. RCGP, London, pp. 12–15.

40 Allery AL, Owen PA and Robling M (1997) Why general practitioners and consultants change their clinical practice: a critical incident study. *BMJ*. **314**: 870–4.

41 Mashru M and Lant A (1997) Interpractice audit of diagnosis and management of hypertension in primary care: educational intervention and review of medical records. *BMJ*. **317**: 942–6.

42 Thomson MA, Oxman AD, Haynes RB *et al.* (1997) Local opinion leaders to improve health professional practice and health care outcomes. In: Bero L, Grilli R, Grimshaw J and Oxman A (eds) *Cochrane Collaboration on Effective Professional Practice Module of The Cochrane Database of Systematic Reviews*. The Cochrane Collaboration, Update Software, Oxford.

43 Lomas J, Anderson GM, Dominick-Pierre K *et al.* (1989) Do practice guidelines guide practice? The effect of a consensus statement on the practice of physicians. *NEJM*. **321**: 1306–11.

44 Costanza ME, Zapka JG, Stoddard AM *et al.* (1991) Physician compliance with mammography guidelines: barriers and enhancers. *J Am Board Fam Pract*. **5**: 143–52.

45 Hyams AL, Brandenburg BA, Lipsitz SR *et al.* (1995) Practice guidelines and malpractice litigation: a two-way street. *Ann Intrn Med*. **122**: 450–5.

46 Burns-Cox CJ (1996) Prevention of blindness: a lost opportunity. *J Med Screening*. **3**: 169.

47 Taplin H (1991) Let guidelines be guidelines. *J Am Board Fam Pract*. **5**: 231–3.

2 The Authority and Validity of Clinical Guidelines

How can a guideline's authority be assessed?

No doctor or court could reasonably depend upon a clinical guideline that has not undergone an adequate development process, which should be evident from a number of key attributes of the guideline, including its:[1,2]

- face credibility
- validity
- reproducibility
- reliability
- representativeness
- clinical applicability
- clinical flexibility
- clarity
- transparency
- scheduled review.

Face credibility

The credibility a guideline commands as a statement of good practice can be termed its *face credibility* or *title to be believed*. This represents the overall credibility accorded to it by relevant user groups: say, in the case of asthma guidelines, by thoracic physicians, GPs and accident and emergency doctors. Different user groups will tend to accord varying degrees of credibility to the same guideline, depending upon their points of view and the relative value they attach to its provenance: guideline development process, its sponsorship, whether it has been rigorously evaluated in practice, and the degree to which leading clinicians in the field have approved and adopted it.

The professional standing of a guideline's developers or sponsors will influence its title to be believed – a guideline created by a Royal College, or sponsored by a specialist medical association will appear to carry greater face credibility than one developed by an unknown group of doctors covering the same clinical area. The title to be believed stems partly from the respect in which the expertise, working practices and values of the guideline authors are held. Guidelines issued by the British Thoracic Society and the British Diabetic Association each individually carry the authority stemming from the manner of their development, and each gains additional authority from the esteem in which their parent bodies are held.[3,4] The Department of Health's decision in 1993 to adopt these guidelines in a drive to improve clinical effectiveness credited the guidelines with an official stamp of approval, superadding an authority which stems from the NHSE's structural and legal position within the NHS.[5]

Dissemination and implementation strategies play a role in enhancing face credibility.[6] The capacity of a guideline sponsoring organization to influence others (perhaps by persuasion, perhaps by incentives) can amplify its apparent authority. It is quite possible for inadequate guidelines to be sponsored and distributed by third parties (for example, the pharmaceutical industry) whose power to influence can be considerable. If a sponsoring body wields power, then whatever the intrinsic merits, an associated guideline is likely to be credited with some of the authority and power of the organization which promulgates it.

But connection between the authority possessed by a developer or sponsor and the true warranty of a guideline is not intrinsic to the guideline itself. The possibility will always exist that an organization might be inappropriately held in high esteem, or that another could lack the expertise required to develop adequate guidelines in specific clinical areas. Since, as we shall see, a guideline's authority can be challenged irrespective of the status of its developer, some independent measure of its authority is required by which to judge how well a guideline's recommendations match valid, relevant research findings, and where lacking, respected medical opinion.

Validity

Guidelines are *valid* if, when correctly followed, they lead to the health gains predicted for them. Guidelines should contain valid statements of recommendation extracted from all relevant high quality medical and scientific evidence, including studies of health care effectiveness. Without an adequate guideline development process advice may emerge that is neither objective nor reproducible. Validity can only be properly gauged through empirical studies which evaluate the effects of guideline adoption and use upon relevant medical process and outcome measures, including effects upon quality of life where relevant.[7,8]

Reproducibility

Were guidelines to be developed concurrently by two or more separate groups of authors covering the same clinical areas, an adequate development process should ensure that substantially the same recommendations emerge from each group, rather than quite different guidance reflecting the subjectivities and experiences of different participants. Where evidence is lacking, or incomplete, this requirement demands that a degree of consensus should exist about clinical management.

Clear and lucid appreciation of available evidence, its strengths and weaknesses, is essential if guideline developers are to reach balanced views on which recommendations can be supported. Possible misreadings and biases can be minimized by adopting explicit criteria with which to appraise research evidence (discussed further below).[9,10] However, as we have seen in Chapter 1, where different groups have set out to produce nationally recognized guidelines covering the diagnosis and management of the same condition using explicit processes to identify and select evidence, a degree of variability in guideline content may nevertheless emerge.[11,12]

In areas where there is little discernible medical consensus, or where it is so patchy that general consensus cannot be achieved using formal methods, resulting clinical guidelines are not likely to be reproducible. From an evidence-based perspective, predominantly opinion-based guidelines run the risk of codifying the customary practices of clinicians who may be unaware of the clinical implications of new research.

Representativeness

Guideline development processes need to balance interests by involving participants representative of the entire domain of practice to be covered by the guideline, including eventual user groups, such as nurses and GPs, and patient organizations. Over representation of one particular group, or the presence of 'persuasive advocates' committed to particular treatments, may result in unwarranted emphasis upon the importance of one set of research findings at the expense of others, or at the expense of every day clinical practices.[9] The possibility clearly exists for serious bias to creep in to guideline development – in the French guidelines programme, major conflicts within guideline development groups have been observed, and formal complaints laid before the Fraud Squad alleging improper conduct by participants.[13]

Participation by representatives of different groups, facilitated sensitively by an independent expert, can help to ensure that consensus embodied in guidelines emanates from a genuine agreement amongst guideline developers, potential users and beneficiaries, and not from agreement forged between a few unrepresentative parties.[4,14,15] Lack of representative input into development can lead to guidelines which, though technically correct, are impractical and inapplicable to the clinical settings for which they are ostensibly designed.

Clinical applicability and clinical flexibility

Clinical applicability refers to the need for guidelines to pertain to significant health problems and specific patient groupings, defined in accordance with scientific, medical and health economic criteria. Identification of valid exceptions to recommendations, and suggestions for how patient preference can be incorporated into clinical decision-making will help to ensure that guidelines allow for appropriate flexibility of application. Tensions which can arise between guidelines, clinical discretion and clinical freedom are discussed in Chapters 5 and 6.

Clarity and reliability

These two attributes refer to different but related properties. The language in which guidance is framed can have a powerful bearing upon the way clinicians view it. *Clarity* demands guidelines be phrased precisely and in clear language. Understanding the scope of a guideline, to which patient populations it is intended to apply and in what particular circumstances, and which particular groups are excluded, depends crucially upon the language in which the guideline is framed. Guideline *reliability* signifies that in the same clinical circumstances, another health professional would interpret and apply the guideline in essentially the same way – a property that depends upon how the guidance is formulated.

Permissive terminology is sometimes thought to protect guideline developers from liability in the event of a directive guideline being associated with injury to a patient. But adoption of non-directive language where directive language is appropriate can attract increased risk for clinician users. Influential commentators have concluded that:

'If drafters conclude that a health care procedure must be performed in certain circumstances but choose to use nondirective language because of concern about legal significance to practitioners who may fail to follow the practice guideline, the practice guideline may, paradoxically, invoke more liability. Use of inappropriately nondirective language may actually mislead practitioners into thinking other approaches are equally appropriate when the evidence indicates otherwise.'[16]

Transparency and scheduled review

Whether guidelines are developed by predominantly opinion-based or evidence-based processes, they should document in their final form the methodology and assumptions used to produce them. To permit users, patients and health care managers properly to assess a guideline's likely value, the experience and qualifications of participating members of the guideline group should be documented, along with a description of the group's working practices. Any peer review and external assessment procedures used in development should be set out, together with how the guidelines were piloted, in which clinical settings, and when review is scheduled.

Guideline development

A variety of approaches to guideline development have been characterized by the Institute of Medicine and the Royal College of General Practitioners.[1,17] Based upon the credibility that can reasonably be accorded to different development strategies, a hierarchy of development strategies has been suggested.[18]

Informal consensus

Recognized or self-appointed, national or local experts may get together to review the medical and scientific evidence for clinical decisions in particular circumstances, producing management guidelines as a result. If the authors of such guidelines do not specify how the evidence was reviewed, what steps were taken to ensure that relevant scientific reports were not inadvertently excluded, do not specify how consensus was reached, or how disagreements were resolved, resulting guidelines are said to be based upon 'informal consensus'.[19]

Such an approach may conceal important differences of opinion within a guideline development group, leading to a 'spurious consensus'.[20] This sort of panel is likely to pool ignorance as well as wisdom.[21] In retelling a story that a US Professor of Health Policy described to him, the editor of the *British Medical Journal* illustrated how 'agreement of the experienced without evidence' can be a poor basis for producing clinical advice. The story concerned an international consensus panel convened for three days per year over five years to develop screening guidelines for the detection of colorectal cancer. At the end of the period, it was reported that:

'... the group recommended a protocol based on regular faecal occult blood tests and sigmoidoscopy. Professor Eddy asked each member of the group then to make a private estimate of how much mortality would be reduced by such a policy; the answers ranged from 0 to almost 100% and were randomly distributed within that range. Yet the consensus had been unanimous. As Hippocrates said, experience is fallacious.'[20]

The point of this story is to recognize that agreement amongst experts can emanate from significantly different understandings and values, and should not be taken as signifying a unitary rationale. Individuals gathered together in committee may come to collective conclusions which individually they may disavow, and consensus can be inappropriately fostered in circumstances of genuine uncertainty and disagreement.[22,23] The *Lancet* reminds us that:

'The clinician unlike the basic scientist has to act even when knowledge is insufficient for a fuller informed decision. A "consensus" view under these circumstances can be achieved in only three ways; by compromise, by selection of an expert panel whose views conform, or by use of language which obscures differences.'[24]

Formal consensus

In contrast to the informal approach, formal and specifiable methods can be adopted to achieve consensus. Using multi-step techniques, systematic reviews of scientific and medical evidence are presented to members of an expert panel who are then required to formulate clinical recommendations, and to modify their recommendations in the light of fellow panellists' formulations. Where criteria of appropriateness have informed this process, and the mechanisms adopted to achieve consensus have been made explicit, resulting guidelines are said to be based upon 'formal consensus'.

But even here, 'consensus' (literally 'joint sense or sympathy') encompasses a wide range of agreements, from active assent, agreement under protest, passive agreement or acquiescence. For these reasons, an American philosopher cautions medical practitioners to 'regard the recommendations of National Institutes of Health consensus development conferences as useful reference tools: not the rulings of philosopher-kings'.[25] For just these reasons, the Evidence-Based Medicine Working Group cautions potential guideline users that:

'Explicit strategies for documenting, describing, and dealing with dissent among judges, or frank reports of the degree of consensus attained, can help you decide whether to adopt or adapt recommendations. Unfortunately, until guideline development methods mature, you will rarely find this information.'[26]

Evidence-based

Efforts to formulate guideline development techniques have been spurred on by attempts to develop evidence-based recommendations. This requires the links between research evidence and guideline recommendations to be made as clear and explicit as possible. Medical and scientific evidence needs first to be systematically assembled using objective search criteria; resulting studies and findings from meta-analyses are then selected for clinical relevance and appropriateness and graded for overall credibility on the basis of the quality of the research, and the clinical significance of the findings. For example, the North of England evidence-based guidelines for *The Primary Care Management of Stable Angina* adopt the evidence grading of the Canadian Task Force Classification, allowing three grades for the quality and significance of evidence:

Level I   Evidence based upon well-designed randomised controlled trials, meta-analyses, or systematic reviews

Level II   Evidence based upon well-designed cohort or case control studies

Level III   Recommendations based upon uncontrolled studies or consensus.

Each recommendation made by the North of England angina guidelines also carries a grading reflecting how strongly the recommendation is anchored in the research evidence:

Grade A   Directly based upon Level I evidence

Grade B   Directly based upon Level II evidence, or, extrapolated recommendation from Level I

Grade C   Directly based upon Level III evidence, or, extrapolated recommendation from Level II.

As Feder and Grimshaw have pointed out, most guidelines, even those which set out to be entirely evidence-based, turn out to be 'hybrids', because they invariably base some recommendations upon an inter-mixture of evidence and opinion.[27] In the North of England angina guidelines, many of the recommendations carry a C grading, and three recommendations had to be based entirely upon a consensus developed within the guideline group because they could not be linked to any research studies. Nevertheless, the advantages of this method include informing potential users about how the development group went about its work, which assumptions it adopted in this task, and how well its recommendations are anchored in research studies of varying rigour.

Other guideline development groups have used variants of these evidence and credibility ratings, depending upon the state of the research evidence for clinical effectiveness. For example, *Guidelines for the Management of Imminent or Actual Violence in Clinical Settings*, developed by the Royal College of Psychiatrists, distinguishes blinded from non-blinded randomized controlled trials and thereby adopts four quality of evidence ratings, whereas in *Guidelines for the Prevention and Treatment of Infection in Patients with an Absent or Dysfunctional Spleen*, the Working Party of the British Committee for Standards in Haematology found that there were no randomized controlled trials or case controlled studies in this clinical area. Their recommendations were simply graded 'A' if based upon published evidence, and 'B' if based upon expert opinion.[28,29]

Assessment of clinical guidelines

Because of concerns that promulgation may confer a false authority not easily distinguishable from real authority, Cluzeau and colleagues have developed a mode of guideline appraisal.[30] Designed particularly for use by professional evaluators or peer reviewers prior to guideline release, it covers guideline development process, content, presentation and applic-ability and poses a series of questions, such as the following:

• Is it clear who was responsible for guideline development?

- Are the objectives of the guideline clearly stated?
- Is the guideline development group adequately described?
- Are the methods adopted to retrieve information upon which to base the recommendations adequately described?
- Are the methods used to interpret the credibility of research studies adequately described?
- How did the guideline development group reach consensus?
- Does the guideline contain an adequate description of the likely costs and benefits of guideline implementation?
- Has the guideline been peer reviewed?
- Will the guideline be regularly reviewed and updated?
- Does the guideline discuss other available guidelines covering the same topic?
- Are there satisfactory descriptions of the scope and applicability of the guideline?
- Is the guideline expressed in unambiguous language?

By answering 46 such questions, an estimate of a guideline's overall worth can be achieved. However, despite growing awareness of the implications for quality of guidance which results from differing guideline development methods, the NHSE remains concerned about the potential for confusion which guideline proliferation could cause, particularly if purchasers adopt poor quality guidelines in specifying health care standards.[31] Whilst viewing guidelines as the responsibility of clinicians (and their professional bodies), the NHSE is keen to support guideline initiatives in areas it judges to be important to the provision of health care nationally. It is therefore commissioning an independent clinical guideline appraisal service with the aim of providing advice on guideline quality. Appraisal is to be 'independent, systematic, transparent, and founded on agreed criteria with objective measurement', and will focus heavily upon guideline development methodology.[32] On the basis of such assessments, the NHSE intends to commend guidelines which meet agreed standards.[33]

There seems little doubt that proliferation of guidelines and their increasing visibility at policy, health authority, practitioner and patient levels means that guideline-driven care will become the expected norm. If commissioning agencies continue to purchase guideline driven health care, patients could be led to expect care of a pre-defined type and quality. Departure from guidelines might then raise suspicions that inferior care had been received fuelling an increase in moves towards litigation. Whether such fears are justified is explored in Chapters 4 and 5.

Summary

The authority of a clinical guideline is easily confused with the medical authority of its authors, developers and sponsors.

Guideline quality is best evaluated by assessing a number of key attributes which determine the true warranty of a guideline.

Several strategies can be used to create clinical guidelines. Each approach has different strengths and weaknesses and may be appropriate in certain circumstances.

References

1 Field M and Lohr K (eds) (1992) *Institute of Medicine Guidelines for Clinical Practice: from development to use.* National Academy Press, Washington DC.

2 Grimshaw J and Russell IR (1994) Achieving health gain through clinical guidelines I: developing scientifically valid guidelines. *Quality in Health Care.* 2: 243–8.

3 British Diabetic Association (1990) *Guidelines for the Development and Integration of General Practitioner Care of Diabetes with Hospital Based Systems.* BDA, London.

4 Statement by British Thoracic Society, British Paediatric Association, Research Unit of the Royal College of Physicians of London, King's Fund Centre, National Asthma Campaign, Royal College of General Practitioners, General Practitioners in Asthma Group, British Association of Accident and Emergency Medicine, and British Paediatric Respiratory Group following a meeting at the Royal College of Physicians, London on 4th & 5th June 1992. Guidelines on the Management of Asthma. *Thorax.* 48: Supplement S1–S24.

5 NHS Management Executive (1993) Improving clinical effectiveness. (EL(93)115). DoH, Leeds.

6 Royal College of General Practitioners (1995) Ensuring that guidelines change clinical practice. In: *The Development and Implementation of Clinical Guidelines.* RCGP, London, pp. 12–15.

7   Grimshaw JM and Russell IT (1993) The effect of clinical guidelines on medical practice: a systematic review of rigorous evaluations. *Lancet.* **2**: 1317–22.

8   NHS Centre for Reviews and Dissemination (1994) Implementing clinical practice guidelines. *Effective Health Care Bulletin.* **8**.

9   Grimshaw JM, Eccles MP and Russell IR (1995) Developing clinically valid practice guidelines. *J Evaluation in Clinical Practice.* **1**: 37–48.

10 Eccles MP, Clapp Z, Grimshaw JM *et al.* (1996) Developing valid guidelines: methodological and procedural issues from the North of England evidence based guideline development project. *Quality in Health Care.* **5**: 44–50.

11 Swales JD (1993) Guidelines on guidelines. *J Hypertension.* **11**: 899–903.

12 Fahey TP and Peters TJ (1996) What constitutes controlled hypertension? Patient based comparison of hypertension guidelines. *BMJ.* **313**: 93–6.

13 Maisonneuve H, Codier H, Durocher A *et al.* (1997) The French clinical guidelines and medical references programme: development of 48 guidelines for private practice over a period of 18 months. *J Evaluation in Clinical Practice.* **3**: 3–13.

14 British Diabetic Association, Research Unit of the Royal College of Physicians, and Royal College of General Practitioners (1993) Report of a Joint Working Party: guidelines for good practice in the diagnosis and treatment of non-insulin dependent diabetes mellitus. *J Roy Col Phys Lond.* **27**: 259–66.

15 Hopkins A (1993) Practice guidelines and bringing the patient into clinical decisions. In: Llewelyn H and Hopkins A (eds) *Analysing How We Reach Clinical Decisions.* Royal College of Physicians of London, London, pp. 117–24.

16 Spernak SM, Budetti PP and Zweig F (1992) *Use of Language in Clinical Practice Guidelines.* Agency for Health Care Policy and Research, Rockville, MD, pp. 1–16.

17 Royal College of General Practitioners (1995) *The Development and Implementation of Clinical Guidelines.* RCGP, London.

18 Woolf SH (1992) Practice guidelines, a new reality in medicine II. Methods of developing guidelines. *Arch Intern Med.* **152**: 946–52.

19 Haines A and Hurwitz B (eds) (1992) *Clinical guidelines: report of a local initiative.* Occasional Paper No. 58. Royal College of General Practitioners, London.

20 Smith R (1991) Where is the wisdom...? The poverty of medical evidence. *BMJ.* **303**: 798–9.

21 Scott E and Black N (1991) When does consensus exist in expert panels? *J Pub Health Med*. **13**: 344.

22 May WE (1985) Consensus or coercion [editorial]. *JAMA*. **254**: 1077.

23 Black D (1997) Corporate tyranny. *J Medical Ethics*. **23**: 269–70.

24 Editorial (1992) *Lancet*. **339**: 1197–8.

25 Tong R (1991) The epistemology and ethics of consensus: uses and misuses of 'ethical' expertise. *J Medicine & Philosophy*. **16**: 409–26.

26 Hayward RSA, Wilson MC, Tunis SR *et al*. for the Evidence-Based Medicine Working Group (1995) Users' guides to the medical literature. *JAMA*. **274**: 570–4.

27 Royal College of General Practitioners (1995) Guideline development. In: *The Development and Implementation of Clinical Guidelines*. RCGP, London, pp. 8–11.

28 Royal College of Pyschiatrists' Clinical Guidelines Programme (1997) *The Management of Violence in Clinical settings: an evidence-based guideline*. RCP, London.

29 Working Party of British Committee for Standards in Haematology, Clinical Haematology Task Force (1996) Guidelines for the prevention and treatment of infection in patients with an absent or dysfunctional spleen. *BMJ*. **312**: 430–4.

30 Cluzeau F, Littlejohns P, Grimshaw J *et al*. (1995) Draft appraisal instrument for clinical guidelines. In: *The Development and Implementation of Clinical Guidelines*. RCGP, London, pp. 23–8.

31 Sutton PA (1996) *Clinical Guidelines Evaluation: final report of the Department of Health guidelines evaluation project*. University of Hull and Royal College of General Practitioners Effective Clinical Practice Programme, Hull.

32 Pink D (Policy Section Head of Clinical Effectiveness, NHSE) (1996) Letter, personal communication.

33 Department of Health (1997) Clinical guidelines and independent appraisal. In: *CMO's Update 16*, p. 8. DoH, London.

3 The Legal Status of Clinical Guidelines

Clinical guidelines can enter the legal arena by two routes. Legislators may use them to assist in the regulation of clinical activities, and the courts may use them in resolution of civil disputes alleging medical negligence. This chapter considers how clinical codes and guidelines interact with legislation (statute law), whilst Chapters 4 and 5 discuss the role guidelines have played, and might yet play, in (case law) actions alleging substandard medical care.

Guidelines backed by statute

Health care systems in several parts of the world appear to be converging in their adoption of guidelines to regulate medical practice. In Europe and the USA statute law has played an important part in these developments. In the UK, greater reliance upon professional self-regulatory mechanisms has meant that there is still a relative paucity of statute in this area, although the situation is now beginning to change. A comprehensive survey of legislation is beyond the scope of this book, but some examples will help to provide an overview of the legal influence which clinical guidelines are beginning to attain.

United Kingdom

In 1990, Parliament established the Human Fertilisation and Embryology Authority (HFEA) to develop and enforce a *Code of Practice* for the proper conduct of health services which use *in vitro* fertilization (IVF) techniques. The *Code* has set and regulated both the ethical and clinical parameters of the provision of IVF in the UK since 1991. It is an elaborate and wide-ranging document covering major areas of clinical practice including the maintenance of scientific and medical standards, clinical and ethical factors to be taken into account when assessing prospective patients seeking fertility treatment, information to be supplied, and counselling to be offered. In accordance with section 26 of the Human Fertilisation and Embryology Act 1990, the *Code* and any subsequent revisions to it, has to be approved by the Secretary of State, who then lays it before Parliament before changes can come into effect.

At its inception, the HFEA announced it would consult widely before deciding what its guidelines should say, recognizing that it faced a 'difficult task of balancing medical, scientific and practical arguments against legitimate public concern'.[1] The Authority's decision to restrict to three the number of fertilized eggs which can be placed in a woman's uterus during treatment by IVF, is a clear example of a guideline emanating from ethical, scientific, safety and cost considerations. Criticized as too restrictive, it nevertheless carries the force of a prescriptive legal rule, having become almost a part of the legal framework itself, though HFEA retains the power to alter it. This particular guideline is unambiguously clear, and its mandatory nature is made clear by enforceable penalties. Non-compliance could result in revocation of the licence required to practise IVF treatment.

Many guidelines adopted or referred to by statutory administrative agencies may not be so clearly defined. For example, the first health promotion programme in general practice, which came into effect in 1992 as a result of statute law, required that patients should be managed clinically 'in line with modern medical opinion and practice guidelines'.[2,3] Regulations spelled out an 'organised programme' of asthma and diabetes care, but also stressed the importance of undefined notions such as 'work[ing] with other professionals when appropriate' and the importance of 'individual management plans' for patient care.[4] As well as being less clearly formulated than the HFEA guidelines, the GP health promotion regulations are also less prescriptive, reflected by the minor consequences which flow from non-compliance – slight loss of income, rather than possible loss of livelihood.

Europe

In France, some 147 mandatory practice guidelines have been introduced under a 1993 statute, Loi Teulade 93–8, covering investigations, prescribing and certain medical procedures. Initially developed by the social security administration responsible for reimbursing private practitioners and the doctors' unions, guideline development has now been taken over by an independent organization, the Agence Nationale pour le Développement de l'Evaluation Médicale. Once published, the guide-lines constitute an enforceable agreement between the social security administration and the doctors.[5,6]

Each set of guidelines is published as a byelaw which also specifies the fines to be applied – up to £2000 – in the event of non-compliance. The 1994 guidelines covering ulcer treatment, for example, stated that there were no grounds for:

- simultaneous prescription of two anti-ulcer drugs
- prescribing a treatment for duodenal ulcer for more than six weeks except when symptoms persist
- prescribing anti-ulcer drugs for chronic gastritis.

Also specified were the levels of fine to be imposed in view of the frequency of guideline transgression by a doctor, and an assumed index of redundancy v iatrogenic harm resulting from non-compliance.

Guidelines come into effect immediately upon publication and enforcement procedures commence after a two month period of obser-vation. In the first two years of the operation of this statute, a survey of 13 000 doctors' prescriptions led to 1278 peer reviews and 186 formal investigations. In 1986, 75 fines were levied.[5-7]

The complex legal position which guidelines may assume is revealed by a Dutch legislative directive which allows doctors intentionally to terminate the lives of their patients only if this is done in accordance with strict guidelines.[8] Drawn-up in association with the Royal Dutch Medical Association, the guidelines pertain to patients suffering from either a physical or psychiatric disorder, and address the following points:

- the request for euthanasia must come only from a competent patient
- the request must be entirely free and voluntary
- the patient's request must be well considered, durable and persistent
- the patient must be experiencing intolerable suffering with no prospect of improvement
- other alternatives to alleviate the patient's suffering must have been considered and found wanting
- euthanasia must be performed by a doctor
- the doctor must consult an independent colleague, before performing euthanasia.

The Dutch directive was put in place in order to formalize a situation that had already evolved through customary medical practice, which over time had gained a degree of support from the courts and from Dutch jurisprudence. The country's penal code, however, remains unchanged; intentional killing of another person continues to be a serious criminal offence carrying a 12-year prison sentence.

Doctors are required to report all cases of euthanasia to the coroner, who then informs the appropriate local magistrate. The magistrate decides whether to prosecute. A doctor faced with prosecution can rely upon strict adherence to the guidelines as providing immunity from being found guilty of murder or manslaughter.[9–12] Any court case would therefore focus upon whether the guidelines had been properly followed, strict adherence constituting an affirmative defence in law.

Despite the immunity provided by the guidelines, under-reporting is probably the rule, with only about 60% of euthanasia cases being notified. Anxiety generated at the prospect of reporting cases where *every* aspect of the guidelines may not have been observed, is thought to be the reason for this level of under-reporting. In an effort to redress the situation, the Dutch government is considering altering the legal arrangements, so that the matter will become the responsibility of regional committees composed of doctors, lawyers and ethicists empowered to exercise discretion in deciding whether the guidelines have been so fundamentally breached as to warrant prosecution.[13]

United States

Statute backed clinical guideline formulation and implementation has probably reached a higher degree of development and sophistication in the USA than in Europe. The range of US legislation in this area is indicated by three separate initiatives.

Peer Review Organizations

One of the first US statutes which attempted to regulate medical practice by using guidelines dates from the 1992 Peer Review Improvement Act, which established Peer Review Organizations (PROs) to ensure the quality and cost-effectiveness of federally funded health care. PROs were empowered by Congress to develop criteria and norms by which to review all Medicare in-patient treatment programmes, and to screen payment claims for evidence of poor quality of care. The criteria have been criticized as insensitive; only a few providers have ever been disqualified from reimbursement because of an elaborate and expensive system of appeals.

Agency for Health Care Policy and Research

The influential Agency for Health Care Policy and Research (AHCPR) was set-up by Congress in 1989 by the Omnibus Reconciliation Act.[14] The Agency was created to commission clinical guidelines covering prevention, diagnosis and clinical management, and was also to conduct research and collect data that would 'enhance the quality, appropriateness, and effectiveness of health care services'.[14,15]

The statute provided for a unit to be established within the AHCPR, entitled The Office of the Forum for Quality and Effectiveness in Health Care (the Forum) charged with arranging for the development and periodic updating of:

'(1) clinically relevant guidelines that may be used by physicians, educators, and health care practitioners to assist in determining how diseases, disorders and health conditions can most effectively and appropriately be prevented, diagnosed, treated, and managed clinically; and

(2) standards of quality, performance measures, and medical review criteria through which health care providers and other appropriate entities may assess or review the provision of health care and assure the quality of such care.'[14]

The Forum, under the leadership of a director, was composed of panels of doctors, patients' representatives and consumers. The Forum was not itself to develop guidelines as these were not intended to become Federal creations, but was 'to arrange' for their development and updating by contracting with public and private organizations such as the American Medical Association and specialist medical and surgical societies. The public policy goal behind its establishment was the introduction of proven cost-effective treatments within a health care system that was increasingly perceived to be too costly and ineffective by international standards.

The Forum's director was empowered to establish the standards and procedures to be followed by guideline contractors, and was also responsible, after the formal adoption of each guideline by the panels, for their dissemination to health care providers, PROs, accreditation agencies, and patient organizations. The Forum was additionally charged to ensure that all adopted guidelines were subsequently evaluated in terms of their impact upon clinical practice.

The Forum's work, and the legislation establishing it, were hailed as a new departure in US health care:

'For the first time, interested parties could turn over their products to a publicly constituted, disinterested body for scrutiny. After appropriate modification, the original guidelines would achieve an imprimatur of sorts from the disinterested body.'[16]

One influential legal scholar has noted that the Forum's panels, which formally adopted and sponsored the guidelines, were designed 'to accommodate and balance the growing interest of a broad range of parties and organizations ... [of] disparate perspectives'.[17] In his view, the legislation was intended to result in clinical guidelines which could be quickly and extensively adopted because they would emerge from *both* impressive medical expertise *and* political consensus. Unfortunately, the Agency's guideline commissioning role was discontinued in 1996, its influence being viewed as too regulatory by a Republican dominated Congress.

The Maine 5-Year Medical Demonstration Project

A five-year experimental project to create legally validated clinical guidelines admissible in court was established by a 1990 statute in Maine, USA, with the aim of establishing:

'standards of practice designed to avoid malpractice claims and increase the defensibility of the malpractice claims that are pursued.'[18,19]

The policy goal behind the legislation is to retain within state boundaries medical specialists such as obstetricians and accident and emergency doctors at high risks of litigation. The process of guideline development adopted was designed by the Maine Medical Association, with the approval of the AHCPR and US national medical and surgical associations. Once guidelines and protocols have been developed, the state Board of Registration can adopt them as rules under Maine's Administrative Procedure Act. If 50% of doctors in the state agree to practise according to the guidelines, then a doctor is empowered to cite the guideline as a complete defence to a medical malpractice claim.

The Maine legislation only allows the guidelines to be cited in a doctor's defence. An aggrieved patient cannot use the fact of a doctor's failure to follow the guidelines as *prima facie* evidence of negligence.[20] This asymmetry between the exculpatory (exonerating) value of guidelines to a doctor, and their lack of inculpatory (implicating) value to a patient may violate the US constitutional requirement of 'due process and equal protection', but this matter has not yet been formally decided upon by US courts.[21]

The legislation establishing the AHCPR guideline programme has had an enormous influence upon the growing discipline of clinical guideline development and evaluation. The Agency was well-funded to commission guidelines based upon methodologically sound processes and upon fundamental reviews of medical practice. The Maine legislation is legally interesting because it suggests that it may not be possible for a doctor to perform negligently if the conduct in question is carried out in accordance with approved guidelines. Although US legal precedent does exist for legislation to influence the standard of care required to avoid liability in negligence,[22] in the UK this would be a matter for the courts to decide upon, on a case by case basis, according to common law principles set out in Chapters 4 and 5.

Summary

Clinical codes and guidelines interact with, and gain backing from, statute law. Examples of such interaction in the UK, Europe and the USA are discussed.

References

1   Human Fertilisation and Embryology Authority (1991) Letter accompanying *Code of Practice*. CH(91)5. HFEA, London.
2   *The National Health Service (General Medical Services) Regulations 1992*. HMSO, London.
3   Department of Health (1993) *The National Health Service Statement of Fees and Allowances*. Para. 30, Sch. 1–3. DoH, Welsh Office, London.
4   Department of Health (1993) *The National Health Service Statement of Fees and Allowances*. Para. 30 Sch. 4, 5. DoH, Welsh Office, London.
5   Durand-Zaleski I, Colin C and Blum-Boisgard C (1997) An attempt to save money using mandatory practice guidelines in France. *BMJ*. 315: 943–6.
6   Maisonneuve H, Codier H, Durocher A *et al*. (1997) The French clinical guidelines and medical references programme: development of 48 guidelines for private practice over a period of 18 months. *J Evaluation in Clinical Practice*. 3: 3–13.

7   Dixon J (1997) France seeks to curb health costs by fining doctors. *BMJ*. **315**: 895–6.

8   Ministry of Justice (1993) *Directie Voorlichting: Act amending Act on the Disposal of the Dead*. Staatsblad, p. 643.

9   Sheldon A (1994) Dutch argue that mental torture justifies euthanasia. *BMJ*. **308**: 431–2.

10 van der Wal G and Dillman RJ (1994) Euthanasia in the Netherlands. *BMJ*. **308**: 1346–9.

11 Walton, Lord (1995) Dilemmas of life and death: Part Two. *J Roy Society Medicine*. **88**: 372–6.

12 van der Wal G, van der Maas PJ, Bosma JM *et al.* (1996) Evaluation of the notification procedure for physician-assisted death in the Netherlands. *NEJM*. **335**: 1706–11.

13 Sheldon A (1997) Dutch euthanasia rules relaxed. *BMJ*. **314**: 325.

14 *US Public Law 101–239, the Omnibus Reconciliation Act 1989*. In: Field M and Lohr K (eds) (1990) *Clinical Practice Guidelines: directions for a new program*. National Academy Press, Washington DC, pp. 107–27.

15 Havighurst C (1990) Practice guidelines for medical care: the policy rationale. *St Louis Univ Law J*. **34**: 777–819.

16 Budetti P (1990) Quoted in Field M and Lohr K (eds) *Clinical Practice Guidelines: directions for a new program*. National Academy Press, Washington DC, p. 26.

17 House of Representatives. Report No. 101–247, 101st Cong., 1st Session (1989) Cited in Havighurst C (1990) Practice guidelines for medical care: the policy rationale. *St Louis Univ Law J*. **34**: 787, ref. 32.

18 Maine Public Law 1990, Ch. 931, 24 MRSA 2972–8. Cited in: Mehlman MJ (1990) Assuring the quality of medical care: the impact of outcome measurement and practice standards. *Law Med Health Care*. **18**: 384, ref. 113.

19 Edwards D (1992) The Maine 5-Year Medical Demonstration Project. Presentation at the Agency for Health Care Policy and Research Conference on Medical Liability Issues. Washington, 1991. Quoted in Field M and Lohr K (eds) *Institute of Medicine Guidelines for Clinical Practice: from development to use*. National Academy Press, Washington DC, p. 130.

20 Smith GH (1993) A case study in progress: practice guidelines and the affirmative defense in Maine. *J Qual Improvement*. **19**: 355–62.

21 Mehlman MJ (1990) Assuring the quality of medical care: the impact of outcome measurement and practice standards. *Law Med Health Care*. **18**: 378.

22 Restatement (Second) of Torts § 285 (1965) Quoted in Schocke-
    moehl G (1984) Admissibility of written standards as evidence of
    the standard of care in medical and hospital negligence actions in
    Virginia. *Univ Richmond LR*. **18**: 737.

4 Clinical Guidelines and Negligence Case Law

Since guidelines are usually developed and implemented with the overall aim of ensuring adequate (if not best) clinical practice, it is understandable that their proliferation might generate medico-legal anxieties.[1,2] This chapter reviews what the courts in the UK have had to say about clinical guidelines on a case by case basis.[3,4] As we shall see, the courts have taken note of guidelines,[5] called for their development and adoption,[6] *over-ruled* prestigious guidelines,[7] and ruled on whether adherence to, or deviation from, specific guidelines was reasonable in particular circumstances.[7-9] Although our focus will be upon cases from the UK, Commonwealth and US cases are touched upon where relevant. Further information concerning legal cases from all these jurisdictions is to be found in Appendix 1.

Lawyers do not generally distinguish between guidelines, protocols or codes of practice and other statements of clinical guidance. Although these instruments differ in ways which may be important to medicine (*see* Chapter 1), in the context of legal proceedings they tend to share the same general significance, since they advise doctors to practise in one way rather than another in particular circumstances, according to a particular clinical standard rather than another.[3]

Negligence

Mention of the word negligence tends to send shivers down medical spines. The *Oxford English Dictionary* defines it as 'a want of attention to what ought to be done or looked after'. The word is potentially applicable to almost any human action, which is said to be negligent if it is judged to have been performed inadequately as compared to a desirable, achievable standard of performance.

To prove negligence in a court of law a plaintiff – the person bringing the action – must show that:

- the defendant doctor owed the plaintiff a *duty of care*, and

- the doctor *breached* this duty of care by failing to provide the *required standard of medical care*, and
- this failure actually *caused* the plaintiff harm.

There are several key terms here which it is useful to elucidate.

Duty of care

Once a doctor–patient relationship clearly exists, the common law holds that doctors have a *duty of care* towards their patients. The nature of this duty was spelt out in 1925 in a case in which a doctor was accused of criminal negligence in performing a traumatic forceps delivery. It was stated then by the trial judge that:

'If a person holds himself out as possessing special skill and knowledge, and he is consulted as possessing such skill and knowledge, by or on behalf of a patient, he owes a duty to the patient to use due caution in undertaking the treatment. If he accepts the responsibility and undertakes the treatment and the patient submits to his discretion and treatment accordingly, he owes a duty to the patient to use diligence, care, knowledge, skill and caution in administering treatment. No contractual relation is necessary, nor is it necessary that the service be rendered for reward.'[10]

If a person has sought advice or treatment which a doctor agrees to provide, then the doctor is obliged to provide reasonable and competent care to the patient. This is the *standard of medical care* required by law.

Breach of duty

The duty of care is imposed by law and its standard is determined by the courts after hearing expert evidence. Since a doctor's duty of care consists of an obligation to provide a fair and reasonable standard of care and competence, breach of this standard consists in providing treatment that falls below such reasonable standard.

Reasonable standard

What is a reasonable standard of care? In UK law the standard of treatment a doctor generally owes to a patient derives from the case of *Bolam v Friern Hospital Management Committee* (1957). In the words of Mr Justice McNair:

'the test is the standard of the ordinary skilled man exercising and professing to have that special skill.'[11]

Doctors are required to act in a manner judged reasonable and proper by a body of other responsible doctors. Judge McNair stated:

'A doctor will not be guilty of negligence if he has acted in accordance with a practice accepted as proper by a responsible body of medical men skilled in that particular art.'[11]

This is what has become known as the 'Bolam test'. Expert testimony helps the courts to ascertain what is accepted and proper practice in specific cases; and this generally ensures that professionally generated standards are applied, rather than standards originating from elsewhere.[12] Although questions of breach of duty are decided primarily on the basis of expert medical evidence, Lord Bridge in another case, *Sidaway* (1985), in applying the Bolam test did not accept that this involved:

'... the necessity "to hand over to the medical profession the entire question of the scope of this duty... including the question of whether there has been a breach of that duty". Of course, if there is a conflict of evidence whether a responsible body of medical opinion approves... in a particular case, the judge will have to resolve that conflict.'[13]

Expert medical evidence is therefore not always conclusive. Courts may examine the substance and rationale of the treatment provided 'not merely the fact that others can be found to support it'.[14] In *Bolitho v City & Hackney Health Authority* (1997), the most recent medical negligence case to reach the House of Lords (which did not feature clinical guidelines), Lord Browne-Wilkinson in the leading judgment stated that:

'the court is not bound to hold that a defendant doctor escapes liability for negligent treatment or diagnosis just because he leads evidence from a number of medical experts who are genuinely of the opinion that the defendant's treatment or diagnosis accorded with sound medical practice... the court has to be satisfied that the exponents of the body of opinion can demonstrate that such opinion has a logical basis. In... cases involving, as they often do, the weighing of risks against benefits, the judge before accepting a body of opinion as being responsible, reasonable or respectable, will need to be satisfied that, in forming their views, the experts have directed their minds to the question of comparative risks and benefits and have reached a defensible conclusion on the matter.'[15]

Causation

Since successful actions in negligence are fault-based, it is essential that the link between fault (breach of duty) and causation of the injuries suffered is firmly established. The proof of causation required in order to recover damages is that the plaintiff is able to show on the balance of probabilities, that the breach of duty caused or materially contributed to injury.[16]

The case of *Early v Newham Health Authority* (1994) illustrates the operation of these concepts and conditions. The plaintiff, a 13-year old girl, alleged that an anaesthetist had employed a faulty protocol during a failed intubation procedure.[9] Prior to elective surgery, it had proved impossible to pass an endotracheal tube during an otherwise routine induction of anaesthesia. The anaesthetist duly followed a protocol adopted in that hospital for such eventualities. This recommended insufflation of the lungs with an oxygen-rich mixture until consciousness was regained. During the course of the procedure the patient awoke whilst still paralysed from suxemethonium, suffering fright and distress as a result. The plaintiff brought an action alleging that the protocol used in her care was substandard.

The doctor and health authority under whose auspices the protocol had been adopted were both charged with negligence. The judge heard evidence about the origins of the protocol, its development and manner of adoption by the division of anaesthesia in the hospital, and was informed of its use in other UK hospitals. Notwithstanding the testimony of a professor of anaesthesia when referring to the protocol, that 'no reasonably competent medical authority would have condoned this drill' the judge found in favour of the defendants. He observed that the authors of this particular protocol had been responsible and competent, neither the doctor nor health authority having been negligent in approving and adopting it.

In *Early* there was no need to formally establish a *duty of care* between anaesthetist and patient because the existence of a relationship of dependence by the patient upon the reasonable skills of the anaesthetist was incontestable. The nub of the case turned on whether there had been a *breach of duty*, a failure by the doctor to provide the *required standard of care*. This was decided by the judge after hearing evidence of the general practices adopted by anaesthetists in this clinical situation, and of the need to balance risks involved in alternative courses of action: such as the risk of transient terror if consciousness is regained against that entailed by adding nitrous oxide to the inspired gas, thereby prolonging anaesthesia until after paralysis has subsided, but at the risk of decreasing the oxygen content of the patient's inspired gases.

Even if breach of duty *had* been found in *Early*, the action in negligence could still have failed if the plaintiff could not also prove, on the balance of probabilities, that the breach in question actually caused the damages complained of. In other words, had it been found that the anaesthetist had adopted a substandard protocol and was thereby in breach of his duty, the next question to be answered would have been 'did the plaintiff suffer physical or psychological damage as a result'? If the answer to this question in these circumstances is 'yes', then the action would be successful and the defendants would be liable for damages. If the answer to this question is 'no' (which would seem unlikely) then despite the finding of a demonstrable breach of duty, the defendants would not be liable for any damages.

The standard of medical care: protocols, guidelines and the law of negligence

The standard of medical care remains one of reasonableness in all the circumstances of the case, and is decided on the basis of an assessment by a judge (or jury in the USA) of evidence which emerges from the testimony of medical experts in the relevant area of practice. The standard of care advocated in written documents including clinical guidelines cannot simply be transcribed into a court setting and used as the legal 'gold standard', by which a judge can decide whether care provided has been substandard. In an important 1967 case in which a patient died as a result of a doctor's failure to enquire about penicillin allergy prior to administering penicillin by injection, the Privy Council (in its judicial role) reiterated that the test of medical negligence is:

'the standard of the ordinary competent practitioner exercising ordinary professional skill, so that evidence from witnesses of the highest professional standing or reference to writings of distinguished medical authorities was not necessary.'[17]

The mere fact that a protocol exists for the care of a particular condition cannot of itself establish that compliance with it would be reasonable in the circumstances, or that non-compliance would be negligent.

Courts are wary of evidence which is not subject to cross-examination, and traditionally view it as hearsay.[18] Protocols or guidelines can be introduced to a UK court by an expert witness as evidence of accepted and customary standards of care, but they cannot be introduced as a *substitute* for expert testimony which can be subjected to examination and cross-examination. The credibility of an expert witness depends to a large extent upon the witness having first-hand experience of the appropriate health care practice.[19] In the *Early* case, the fact that the plaintiff's main expert witness was a retired anaesthetist of high academic rank, may have been a factor counting against the relevance of his testimony to current practice. The trial judge clearly was satisfied that the protocol which the anaesthetist followed had been one accepted by a responsible body of other anaesthetists. In these circumstances, the judge could only have found it substandard if it nevertheless constituted obvious folly by exposing patients to unjustified risk (a possible situation that is discussed further below).

The Privy Council judgment of 1967 emphasized that the appropriate standard of medical care is neither best practice, nor the practice of 'super specialists' unless that is the type of care that is under scrutiny.[18] Judgment in the Bolam case referred to doctors 'skilled in that particular art' and in subsequent legal cases these words have been understood to mean that the standard of care required from one sort of practitioner could be different from that required from another.[17,20] Lord Bridge reiterated this point in 1985 in his House of Lords judgment in the case of *Sidaway v Governors of Bethlem Royal Hospital*:

'The language of the *Bolam* test clearly requires a different degree of skill from a specialist in his own field than from a general practitioner.'[21]

We have seen that the standard of medical care required in law is that of reasonable care in the appropriate circumstances, and that the courts' view on this is formed on a case by case basis after hearing and examining what a body of responsible doctors believes to be reasonable and proper in the circumstances. This is a broadly expressed standard. Its strength lies in allowing well founded co-existence of differences of medical opinion as to what constitutes appropriate treatment in particular circumstances, where the practice of medicine, some argue, can be characterized 'as much an art as a science'.[22] The test allows for professional differences of opinion and for the possibility that two or more schools of medical thought may co-exist about how a patient should be treated in a particular situation. As one judge has observed:

'In the realm of diagnosis and treatment there is ample scope for genuine difference of opinion and one man is not negligent merely because his conclusion differs from that of other professional men.'[23]

The same point was made in the case of *Maynard v West Midlands Regional Health Authority* (1985), where a Law Lord ruled that:

'a judges' preference for one body of distinguished professional opinion to another also professionally distinguished is not sufficient to establish negligence in a practitioner whose actions have received the seal of approval of those whose opinions, truthfully expressed, honestly held, were not preferred... For in the realm of diagnosis and treatment negligence is not established by preferring one respectable body of professional opinion to another. Failure to exercise the ordinary skill of a doctor (in the appropriate speciality, if he is a specialist) is necessary.'[24]

There is probably little legal basis, therefore, to the anxiety expressed by some, that clinical guidelines might cause one group of doctors to be judged in court by inappropriate standards of care laid down by an entirely different group.[25,26] Health care evaluation studies can usefully contribute to greater clarity on this matter, particularly if they focus upon the mismatch between the clinical experiences of guideline developers, the guidelines they generate and clinicians' practices. One research group on the management of back pain recently concluded that:

'If general practitioners are going to use guidelines they must be satisfied that the guidelines are based on good evidence gathered in primary care and applied sensibly in that setting.'[27]

In the USA, it has been claimed that clinical guidelines and protocols offer a better chance for defendant doctors to be held to consensual standards of diagnosis and treatment, than do insufficiently tested idiosyncratic standards put forward as customary by expert witnesses.[28] By supplying 'guideline norms', the argument goes, clinical guidelines could help judges and juries to be more consistent when coming to a decision as to what kinds of care constitute negligence.

Similar concerns about the neutrality of expert witnesses have arisen in the UK, but with quite different solutions being proposed.[29] These include greater transparency and disclosure to both sides of a legal action, of communications between lawyers and witnesses about pretrial meetings between expert witnesses, and of the possible appointment of an agreed joint expert witness to both sides of a dispute on occasion.[30]

Can adherence to guidelines protect doctors from liability?

An instance in which the highest UK court found that guidelines drawn-up by a responsible body of opinion can offer a degree of protection to clinicians in the eyes of the law is to be found in the case of Tony Bland (1993), a victim of the Hillsborough football stadium disaster.[31] The guidelines in question, developed by the Medical Ethics Committee of the British Medical Association after wide-ranging consultation, were safeguards to be observed before discontinuing artificial nutrition and hydration to patients in persistent vegetative state (PVS).[32, 33] Lord Goff, in one of the leading judgments, stated that:

'study of this document left me in no doubt that, if a doctor treating a PVS patient acts in accordance with the medical practice now being evolved by the Medical Ethics Committee of the BMA, he will be acting with the benefit of guidance from a responsible and competent body of professional opinion, as required by the *Bolam* test.'[31]

Although the *Bland* case was not a case involving an action in negligence, according to this judgment the BMA guidelines constituted the appropriate Bolam test in the clinical circumstances, because they amounted to 'guidance from a responsible body of professional opinion'. Since this is the standard of care required by law, compliance with these guidelines was also compliance with the law. However, the Law Lords clearly felt that simple compliance with the guidelines, given the moral complexity and potential public concern about decisions of this sort, did not provide sufficient grounds for all such subsequent clinical decisions; and they ruled that future proposals to withdraw nutrition and hydration from patients in PVS should first come before the courts for approval.

The effect of the judgment in the *Bland* case was to ensure that the doctors and health authority would not face a legal action alleging negligence if Tony Bland's treatment was to be discontinued. Although adherence to the BMA guidelines was deemed to provide legal protection, the court did not dissect out which aspects of the guidelines it viewed as mandatory and which it viewed as more permissive. The judgment recognized that guidance was 'being evolved', which implies an appreciation by the courts that the required standard of care is likely to change over time. Clinicians are known to hold differing views on

PVS management and differing interpretations of the current legal requirements, and subsequent court decisions have hinted at a degree of flexibility in guideline interpretation.[34] In *Frenchay Healthcare NHS Trust v S* (1994), for example, the diagnosis of PVS had been confirmed after only four months, but this was not viewed by the Court of Appeal as a material deviation from the required standard of care, even though the BMA guidelines recommend that the diagnosis should not be viewed as properly established until 12 months after injury.[35]

In the case of *W v Edgell* (1989), an action for breach of confidence, the first judge did not accept that Dr Edgell's disclosure of his assessment of W was a legally culpable breach of confidence.[36] W, who had killed four people, had subsequently been convicted of manslaughter on the grounds of diminished responsibility. He was detained in a secure hospital, and sought an injunction against the Home Secretary and others to prevent them disclosing or using a report prepared by Dr Edgell at the request of W's solicitors. The report was unfavourable towards W in his application to a mental health tribunal to be considered for discharge or transfer to a regional secure unit. On receipt of Edgell's report, W's solicitors had withdrawn his application to the tribunal.

Dr Edgell had been asked to examine W solely to provide the patient and his solicitors with his own assessment. Without W's permission, Edgell sent a copy of his report to the hospital in which W was detained. The hospital subsequently forwarded the report to both the Home Secretary and the tribunal. W claimed that Dr Edgell had breached his duty of confidentiality towards him. The judge at first instance, Judge Scott, found that the circumstances of the case fell squarely within the General Medical Council's (GMC) guidelines (which were referred to as 'rules' in the judgment). The GMC guidelines on this subject laid out in the then current 'Blue Book', *Advice on Standards of Professional Conduct and Medical Ethics*, specifically stated that doctors were permitted to disclose confidential medical information to other doctors bearing clinical responsibility for a patient without that patient's permission.

General Medical Council guidelines generally connote more than mere advice, to be heeded or not at a doctor's discretion, since the GMC is a statutory body which wields disciplinary powers.[37] In this case, the courts had to decide whether adherence to guidelines on the ethics of medical practice conferred legal protection. Judge Scott's view was affirmed by the Court of Appeal, which accepted that the GMC's written guidelines correctly specified legally valid exceptions to the duty of confidence owed by a doctor to a patient.[38]

Does deviation from guidelines constitute negligence?

That deviation from professionally accepted and well-established guidelines may increase exposure to liability in medical negligence is a concern often voiced by clinicians. The legal significance of deviation from standard practice was enunciated in a key judgment by Lord Clyde, in *Hunter v Hanley* (1955).[23] The case related to injuries a patient had sustained from an injection:

'... in regard to allegations of deviation from ordinary professional practice ... such a deviation is not necessarily evidence of negligence. Indeed, it would be disastrous if this were so, for all inducement to progress in medical science would be destroyed. Even a substantial deviation from normal practice may be warranted by the particular circumstances.'[23]

Three facts require to be proven, he reiterated, in order to establish liability in the case of a doctor accused of negligence as a result of deviating from normal practice:

'... First of all it must be proved that there is a normal practice; secondly it must be proved that the defendant has not adopted that practice; and thirdly (and this is of crucial importance) it must be established that the course the doctor has adopted is one which no professional man of ordinary skill would have taken if he had been acting with ordinary care.'[23]

Summarizing the case of *Loveday v Renton and Wellcome Foundation Ltd* (1990), the editor of *Medical Law Reports* explained that the court held *obiter** that failure to observe particular contraindication guidelines when administering whooping cough vaccination:

'would not in itself constitute negligence because there was a respectable and responsible body of medical opinion that some contraindications should not be observed because the risk of disease outweighed any actual or possible risk from the vaccine.'[8]

The case concerned a baby girl who suffered brain damage after receiving pertussis vaccination, despite coming within the then

---

* *Obiter* here means that this particular reasoning was not central to the main issues which the court had to decide in this case, namely whether whooping cough vaccine could cause brain damage, and if so, whether the doctor acted negligently in this particular case.

current contraindications issued by the Department of Health. The judgment is interesting for its explication of the relationship between guidelines, expert testimony, and the opinions of other respectable authorities:

'... In so far as the plaintiff seeks to rely on the contraindications as evidence of the opinions of experts not called as witnesses that the vaccine can cause brain damage, this evidence is inadmissible in law. The reason for this is obvious; it is not known who holds the opinion or basis of it; and the evidence is not tested in cross-examination before the court. It is hearsay. But it is part of the medical literature in the case, experts are entitled to and have commented on it ...

The question of whether the vaccine can cause brain damage is not answered by showing that there is a respectable and responsible body of medical opinion that the vaccine can, albeit rarely, cause permanent brain damage, or that this view may be more widely held than the contrary... The works of learned and qualified authors form part of the general corpus of medical and scientific learning on the subject and can be relied upon and adopted by suitably qualified experts. These experts may have their opinions tested in the light of this literature.'

Even had it been possible to establish in the *Loveday* case that pertussis vaccine *could* cause brain damage (which the case left unproved), the judge clearly believed that the third and crucial condition set out in the earlier case of *Hunter v Hanley* could not be established, despite the breach of official Department of Health guidelines, namely that the course the doctor adopted was one which 'no professional man of ordinary skill would have taken if he had been acting with ordinary care'.[23]

So long as customary care sets the legal standard of care, mere deviation from a guideline would be unlikely to be accepted as evidence of negligence by a UK court, as long as the particular deviation accorded with an approved practice recognized by a responsible body of doctors; or unless, after a careful explanation as to why non-standard treatment represented the best option in the circumstances, the patient had consented to innovatory treatment. The judge in the *Bolam* case stated that:

'in the case of a medical man negligence means failure to act in accordance with the standards of reasonably competent medical men at the time. That is a perfectly accurate statement, as long as it is remembered that there may be one or more perfectly proper standards.'[11]

The 1990 case of *Cranley v Medical Board of Western Australia*, which involved alleged misconduct by an Australian GP further illustrates the importance the common law usually attaches to the existence of more than two schools of thought. In prescribing injectable diazepam to heroin addicts, Dr Cranley had deviated from the Australian *National Methadone Guidelines* and, as a consequence, he was found guilty of 'infamous and improper conduct'. But the Supreme Court of Western Australia upheld his appeal when it heard of a minority medical opinion in Australia which supported treatment of opiate addicts as Dr Cranley had done, within a harm reduction framework.[39]

Lack of professional consensus

Where professional consensus towards a clinical situation is lacking, courts may be influenced by a dominant view advocated by existing guidelines, such as occurred in the initial stages of *Cranley v Medical Board of Western Australia*. In a similar case in the UK, *Dally v GMC* (1987), Dr Dally stood accused of serious professional misconduct in her prescribing of methadone, and in failing to follow 'guidelines laid down for good clinical practice'.[40]

The GMC is not a court of law but a tribunal of the medical profession established by statute. Although Dr Dally was not found guilty of misconduct on account of breaching the guidelines, she believed that the hearing had been brought against her because she had dissented from a prevailing 'establishment' view on how, at that time, drug addicts should be treated. She later commented:

'In medicine, guidelines drawn up by the establishment are all too easily converted into regulations and a means of punishing dissenters.'[41]

Dr Dally's harm reduction approach to the treatment of opiate addicts had not accorded with the policy recommended by Dangerous Drug Units, nor with the 1984 Department of Health guidelines,[42] though her approach has since gained greater official credibility. The legal scholar and historian of the GMC, Russell Smith, agrees with her assessment. In the case of *Dally v GMC*, he argues:

'One was left with the unhappy situation of a doctor having her conduct adjudicated and its undesirability declared, presumably for the benefit of the whole medical community in knowing what was acceptable conduct in the eyes of the GMC, when she had merely been following one school of thought which had its own substantial body of advocates.'[43]

If the courts allowed a dominant school of thought to set the standard of care required to avoid a charge of negligence (which was not, in fact, what Dr Dally stood accused of), then an undesirable uniformity of medical care could be the result. In the area of negligence, a minority view will not normally be rejected by the courts if it is supported by a responsible body of doctors.[44] To quote once again from Judge McNair in the influential *Bolam* case:

'a doctor is not negligent... merely because there is a body of opinion that takes a contrary view.'[11]

The Bolam test is sometimes called the customary care standard. It can be understood as representing an aggregate of individual clinical judgments informed by scientific evidence and professional experience; this sets the expected norm. Its advantages are that it takes account of evolving standards of medical care. Though legally imposed, it is a professionally derived standard; it allows for differences of opinion, and is sufficiently broadly expressed to encompass a variety of medical opinions about specific clinical scenarios.[13]

However, the Bolam test appears to be a 'state of the art' descriptive test about what *is* done in practice, rather than a normative one about what *ought* to be done. In other words, it may be thought to demand too little to encourage higher standards of care, and to licence any treatments which a body of responsible practitioners testify should be adopted in circumstances similar or identical to that before the court.

Nevertheless, the law of negligence does not necessarily assume that the medical profession is reasonable and responsible in its creation and adoption of customary medical procedures. The American jurist, Oliver Wendell Holmes, aptly stated the legal position in 1903 when he wrote:

'What usually is done may be evidence of what ought to be done... but what ought to be done is fixed by a standard of reasonable prudence, whether it is complied with or not.'[45]

As another US judge put it:

'Courts must in the end say what is required; there are precautions so imperative that even their universal disregard will not excuse their omission.'[46]

The courts can find health care professionals negligent despite hearing from expert witnesses that they themselves would have adopted the practice under scrutiny in similar circumstances.[47] But this generally only occurs in cases where customary practices have appeared to place patients at risk in situations where an alternative course of action exists which is clearly less risky, where the courts find what they term 'obvious folly'.[48]

In the case of the Bolam test, who should decide by what criteria what constitutes 'a responsible body of medical men skilled in that particular art' seems insufficiently clearly specified. There remain, Ian Kennedy has argued, unresolved tensions in UK common law concerning answers to such questions:

'In its crudest form, the question asked is whether, when challenged as to his practice, a defendant doctor can merely call together a group of friends and colleagues who share his views, assert that they are, by that token, "a responsible body of medical men", and thereby prevent the plaintiff carrying the burden of proof... At a deeper level, more subtle questions arise as to how application of this test can allow the law to distinguish, for example, between a group of rogue practitioners, a group of unorthodox practitioners and a group of eminently respectable (if orthodox) practitioners engaged in treatment... But is it the role of the court merely to sit back and say a practice is responsible if those who practise it say it is? If it is, then *Bolam* remains ascendant. If it is not, then the culture reflected by *Bolam* can no longer survive.'[49]

In other common law countries, the value of the Bolam test is being questioned.[50] In Australia, the Supreme Court emphasized in 1995 that:

'It is not the law that if all or most of the medical practitioners in Sydney habitually fail to take an available precaution to avoid foreseeable risk of injury to the patients that none can be found guilty of negligence.'[51]

Another distinguished Australian Judge has expressed the view, non-judicially, that the Bolam test may well be:

'a hang-over from the Victorian age when Nanny was supposed to "know best"... arising from the class system and the hierarchical nature of English society and reflecting the unwillingness of one profession (the law, represented by the judge) to countenance ordinary people challenging the rules laid down by another profession (medicine).'[52]

In UK cases too, judges have noted that a major disadvantage of Bolam is that it gives too much power to the medical profession which, it is argued, should not be allowed to validate its own practices in court.[53]

Guideline-informed standards of care

The main justification for judicial reliance upon customary care standards has been the belief that medical technical matters, particularly in the realm of diagnosis and treatment, are beyond the knowledge and expertise of judges and lay people, and are therefore best left to 'experts'. Could widespread adoption of clinical guidelines begin to undermine this justification? Guidelines can offer doctors, patients and purchasers explicit examples of standards of care for use in specific clinical circumstances. Such guidelines could be thought to do away with the need for expert testimony in a court of law's quest to define the legal standard of care, because the court could have direct access to the appropriate standard from a clinical guideline. One academic health lawyer has foreseen just such a possibility:

'Just as clinical guidelines may help to demystify clinical decision-making for managers and purchasers, they may have a similar effect on English judges. If clinical decision-making can be reduced to a series of steps outlined in a published guideline, the argument would go, it must also be susceptible of similar elucidation in court. This of itself could lead to a greater willingness in English judges to assess for themselves the reasonableness of clinical practice rather than simply asking whether the defendant's clinical management as a whole was acceptable to a responsible body at the time.'[54]

There are as yet few clear cut cases in which this possibility has been translated into legal proceedings in the UK, but in one such case, *Sutton v Population Family Planning Programme Ltd* (1981), a nurse who failed to follow the prescribed procedure for referring a patient with a breast lump was on that account found negligent.[55]

If clinical guidelines were to become widely and pervasively adopted as the Government has signalled they will, then guideline-informed care might come to be viewed by the courts as sufficient evidence of the customary norm.[56] In such a situation, departure from guideline approved-care might be viewed as *prima facie* evidence of a case to answer. The possibility of such a scenario has not escaped the notice of health lawyers:

'While it is extremely unlikely that the existence of protocols will lead to the elimination of the *Bolam* test altogether, there could be a strong argument for reversing the burden of proof in cases where guidelines are not followed. A doctor who had decided not to follow the definitive guidelines produced by experts in his field would be required to justify his decision. He could call upon expert witnesses to assist him, but the burden of proof would be on him and not the patient.'[57]

The effects of any such changes in legal emphasis could well be to encourage adherence to clinical guidelines and therefore, perhaps, the development of unthinking conformity (*see* Chapter 6). But this would come into tension with another thread of the common law which views the essence of medical practice to be the exercise of professional judgment and clinical discretion, the subject of the next chapter.

Summary

The standard of medical care required by law is decided on a case by case basis on the evidence which emerges from the testimony of medical experts in the relevant area of practice. Guidelines are regarded by the courts as hearsay evidence only. Standards of care advocated in written documents, including clinical guidelines, cannot therefore be used as the legal 'gold standard' to decide whether care provided has been substandard.

Nevertheless, protocols or guidelines can be introduced to a UK court by an expert witness but not as a *substitute* for expert testimony.

The mere fact that a protocol or guideline exists for the care of a particular condition does not of itself establish that compliance with it would be reasonable in the circumstances, or that non-compliance would be negligent.

As guideline-informed health care increasingly becomes customary, so acting outside the guidance of guidelines could expose doctors to the possibility of being found negligent, unless they can prove a special justification in the circumstances.

References

1   Harvey I and Roberts C (1987) Clinical guidelines, medical litigation, and the current medical defence system. *Lancet.* i: 145–7.

2   Cotton P, Ross S and Sullivan F (1996) *Guidelines and Practice-based Protocol Development: the involvement and attitudes of general practitioners and practice nurses*. University Department of General Practice, Glasgow, pp. 1–8.

3   Hurwitz B (1994) Clinical guidelines: proliferation and medico-legal significance. *Quality in Health Care*. 3: 37–44.

4   Hurwitz B (1995) Clinical guidelines and the law: advice, guidance or regulation? *J Evaluation in Clinical Practice*. 1: 49–60.

5   Re A and others (minors) (child abuse: guidelines) (1991) 1 *WLR*: 1026–32.

6   Re F (mental patient: sterilization) (1989) 2 *WLR*: 1025–62.

7   Re W (a minor) (1992) 3 *WLR*: 758–82.

8   Loveday v Renton and Wellcome Foundation Ltd (QBD) (1990) 1 *Med LR*: 117–204.

9   Early v Newham Health Authority (1994) 5 *Med LR*: 214–17.

10 R v Bateman (1925) Quoted in: Kennedy I and Grubb A (1994) *Medical Law: text and materials*. Second ed. Butterworths, London, p. 400.

11 Bolam v Friern Hospital Management Committee (1957) 2 *All ER*: 118–28 at 122.

12 Lord Scarman (1987) Law and medical practice. In: Byrne P (ed.) *Medicine in Contemporary Society*. King Edward's Hospital Fund for London, London, p. 132.

13 Sidaway v Board of Governors of the Bethlem and the Maudsley Hospital (House of Lords) (1985) 1 *All ER*: 643–66.

14 Newdick C (1995) *Who Should We Treat?* Clarendon Press, Oxford, p. 86.

15 Bolitho v City & Hackney Health Authority (1997) 3 *WLR*: 1151–61 at 1159.

16 Kennedy I and Grubb A (1989) *Medical Law: text and materials*. Butterworths, London, pp. 426–46.

17 Chin Keow v Government of Malaysia (Privy Council) (1967) 1 *WLR*: 813–17 at 813H.

18 Howard M and Crane P (1982) *Phipson on Evidence*. Sweet & Maxwell, London, p. 562.

19 Hodgkinson T (1990) *Expert Evidence: law and practice*. Sweet & Maxwell, London, p. 137.

20 Wilsher v Essex Area Health Authority (1987) Quoted in: Kennedy I and Grubb A (1989) *Medical Law: text and materials*. Butterworths, London, p. 400.

21 Sidaway v Bethlem Royal Hospital Governors and others (1985) 1 *All ER*: 660.

22   Newdick C (1995) *Who Should We Treat?* Clarendon Press, Oxford, p. 82.

23   Hunter v Hanley. Session Cases 200–8 (Court of Session) (1955) Quoted in: Kennedy I and Grubb A (1989) *Medical Law: text and materials.* Butterworths, London, p. 420.

24   Maynard v West Midlands Regional Health Authority (1985) 1 *All ER*: 635–42.

25   Farmer A (1993) Medical practice guidelines: lessons from the United States. *BMJ*. 307: 313–17.

26   Gray DP (1992) Editor's preface. In: Haines A and Hurwitz B (eds) (1992) *Clinical guidelines: report of a local initiative.* Occasional Paper No. 58, p. vii. RCGP, London.

27   Little P, Smith L, Cantrel E *et al.* (1996) General practitioners' management of acute back pain: a survey of reported practice compared with clinical guidelines. *BMJ*. 312: 485–8.

28   Kinney ED and Wilder MM (1989) Medical standard setting in the current mal-practice environment: problems and possibilities. *22 Univ of Cal at Davis Law Review*: 421.

29   Shepard RT (1991) Expert evidence. *Medico-Legal Journal*. 59/1: 67–8.

30   Medical Negligence Working Group (1995) *Lord Woolf's Inquiry: access to justice. Medical negligence litigation consultation paper.* Medical Negligence Working Group, London, pp. 24–8.

31   Airedale NHS Trust v Bland (Guardian *ad litem*) (1993) 1 *All ER*: 821–96.

32   Medical Ethics Committee of the British Medical Association (1992) *Discussion Paper on Treatment of Patients in Persistent Vegetative State*. BMA, London.

33   British Medical Association (1993) *Guidelines on Treatment Decisions for Patients in Persistent Vegetative State*. BMA, London.

34   Grubb A, Walsh P, Lambe N *et al.* (1996) Survey of British clinicians' views of patients in persistent vegetative state. *Lancet*. 348: 35–40.

35   Frenchay Healthcare NHS Trust v S (Court of Appeal) (1994) 2 *All ER*: 403–13.

36   W v Edgell (1989) 1 *All ER*: 1089–109.

37   The General Medical Council (1993) *Professional Conduct and Discipline: fitness to practise*. GMC, London.

38   Judge Scott's judgment on this point was affirmed by Sir Stephen Brown in the Court of Appeal. Lord Justice Bingham had some reservations about whether in fact Edgell's relationship to W did

fall within the exception stated in para. 81(b) because he did not believe that Edgell's relationship to W could correctly be described as 'having a continuing and professional relationship with the patient'. See W v Edgell (Court of Appeal) (1990) 9 *WLR*: 474–93 at 485G, 489G, 489H.

39 Cranley v Medical Board of Western Australia (Sup Ct WA) (1992) 3 *Med LR*: 94–113.

40 Dally v General Medical Council (Privy Council) (1987) *Lexis transcript*. Mead Data Central, OH.

41 Dally A (1990) *A Doctor's Story*. Macmillan, London, pp. 127, 164.

42 Department of Health (1984) *Guidelines of Good Clinical Conduct in the Treatment of Drug Misuse*. DoH, Welsh Office, London.

43 Smith RG (1994) *Medical Discipline: the professional conduct jurisdiction of the General Medical Council, 1858–1990*. Clarendon Press, Oxford, p. 71.

44 Defreitas v O'Brien (1995) *Times*. February 16.

45 Quoted in: Kinney ED and Wilder MM (1989) Medical standard setting in the current malpractice environment. **22** *Univ of Cal at Davis Law Review*: 423, footnote 98, citing Texas & Pacific Railway v Behymer (1903), **189** *US*: 468, 470.

46 The words of Justice Hand quoted in: Helling v Carey (1974) **519** *Pacific Reporter 2d Series*: 981.

47 Holyoak J (1990) Raising the standard of medical care. *Legal Studies*. **10**: 201–11.

48 See for example, the cases of Anderson v Chasney (1949), Hucks v Cole (1968) and Clarke v Adams (1950) quoted in Kennedy I and Grubb A (1989) *Medical Law: text and materials*. Butterworths, London, pp. 414–17.

In the Canadian case of Anderson v Chasney, which involved a retained swab after operation, the Court of Appeal of Manitoba received expert testimony to the effect that it was not usual practice routinely to count swabs prior to completion of an operation in some hospitals. However, the Court decided:

'Whether or not it is negligence to omit... to have a count kept is not a matter which requires an expert to decide... If a practitioner refuses to take an obvious precaution, he cannot exonerate himself by showing that others also neglect to take it.'

In Hucks v Cole, a doctor who caused serious injury as a result of failing to treat a septicaemic patient with penicillin was held to have been negligent despite expert testimony that the defendant doctor had acted in accordance with an approved practice. In the Court of Appeal, Sachs LJJ stated:

'When the evidence shows that a lacuna in professional practice exists by which risks of grave danger are knowingly taken... and the Court finds that... in the light of current professional knowledge, there is no proper basis for the lacuna, and that it is definitely not reasonable that those risks should have been taken, its function is to state that fact and where necessary to state that it constitutes negligence. In such a case the practice will no doubt thereafter be altered to the benefit of patients.'

49   Kennedy I (1995) Negligence: breach of duty. Responsible body of opinion. 3 *Med Law Review*: 195–8.
50   Helling v Carey (1974) **519** *Pacific Reporter 2d Series*: 981–5.
51   Albrighton v Royal Prince Alfred Hospital (1980) **2** *NSWLR*: 542 (CA), 562. Quoted in: Kirby M (1995) Patients' rights – why the Australian courts have rejected 'Bolam'. *J Medical Ethics*. 21: 5–8.
52   Kirby M (1995) Patients' rights – why the Australian courts have rejected 'Bolam'. *J Medical Ethics*. 21: 5–8.
53   Donaldson J. In: Sidaway v Board of Governors of Bethlem Royal Hospital (Court of Appeal) (1984) 1 *All ER*: 1018–36.
54   Stern K (1995) Clinical guidelines and negligence liability. In: Deighan M and Hitch S (eds) *Clinical Effectiveness: from guidelines to cost-effective practice*. Earlybrave Publications Ltd, Brentwood, pp. 127–35.
55   Sutton v Population Family Planning Programme Ltd (Unreported) (1981) Cited in: Montgomery J (1977) *Health Care Law*. Oxford University Press, Oxford, p. 183.
56   Secretary of State for Health (1997) *The New NHS* (Cmnd 3807). HMSO, London.
57   Harpwood V (1994) NHS reform, audit, protocols and standards of care. *Medical Law International*. 1: 241–59.

5 Guidelines, Author Liability and Clinical Discretion

The Bolam test of the standard of clinical care has come under pressure in the past two decades. But it seems unlikely to be superseded in the UK in the near future, by a standard of care which the courts determine without reference to a responsible body of medical practitioners. Expert witnesses in court, as representatives of a responsible body of practitioners, will almost certainly be required to provide testimony about the standards of care they judge to be reasonable in the circumstances.[1]

In looking to clinical guidelines for evidence of standards of care, courts may experience difficulty in deciding whether guidelines:

- set out minimum reasonable standards, or
- codify customary standards, or
- recommend best practice.

A distinguished Canadian lawyer has reminded us that courts need to distinguish 'ideal medical care from reasonable care'.[2] To illustrate, the 1993 version of the British Thoracic Society's guidelines on the treatment of asthma recommended inhaled cromoglycate be used in the first step of a treatment ladder for 'nearly all' children. But a random sample of 100 general paediatricians sent a questionnaire enquiring about their treatment approaches to asthma in 1995 (90% response rate) showed that 79% deviated from this advice, omitting cromoglycate altogether and commencing inhaled steroids at an earlier stage than recommended by the guidelines. The authors of the study concluded that when:

'audit shows a gap between protocol and practice then either the guidelines or the practice or both, should change... The British Thoracic Society's guidelines should be changed to match more closely what paediatricians do.'[3]

Leaving aside which approach to the treatment of childhood asthma is safer and more cost-effective, courts are likely to accept that an established approach to treatment, even if adopted by a minority of doctors, would be likely to constitute a reasonable standard of care, so long as the minority opinion was a responsible one. The most recent version of the British Thoracic Society's guidelines has moved some way towards the customary practice revealed by the questionnaire, now recommending *either* inhaled steroids or inhaled sodium cromoglycate as first line prophylaxis to children with asthma aged under five.[4]

When the pace of research and development within health care was considerably less than it is now, an early standard text on medical negligence advised that:

'The practitioner who treads the well worn path... will usually be safer, as far as concerns legal liability, than the one who adopts a newly discovered method of treatment. *[Doctors]* ought not in general to resort to a new practice or remedy until its efficacy and safety had been sufficiently tested by experience.'[5]

An important judgment supporting this view stated that:

'A doctor might not be negligent if he tried a new technique but if he did he must justify it before the Court. If his novel or exceptional treatment had failed disastrously he could not complain if it was held that he went beyond the bounds of due care and skill as recognized generally.'[6]

This judgment, handed down in 1961 in the case of *Landau v Werner* has been influential in protecting the public from inadequately evaluated innovatory therapy. However, the modern Health Service has adopted an increasingly strong research and development orientation that values rapid research implementation. Clinical guidelines which aim to bring the results of research to the patient by directly influencing clinicians, rather than by waiting for research findings to percolate through the profession, are now under intensive development.

The evolution of the asthma guidelines highlights tensions which can obtain between the value guidelines accord to customary care practices, and how much guidelines may be created with the aim of changing current practices. Some guidelines do not, in fact, aim to reflect a customary standard of care at all. Indeed, an important rationale for their introduction acknowledges that customary care may be insufficiently evidence-based. Guideline dissemination in these circumstances aims to move customary care towards 'higher' evidence-based standards. Such guidelines are designed to hasten the incorporation of research findings into routine practice.[7]

The rationale is well-stated by the US Evidence-Based Working Group:

'To the extent that clinicians rely on community standards or opinion leaders to guide their practice, there is an implicit assumption that their needs for information are being met through these means, i.e. that community standards and the recommendations of experts (opinion leaders) reflect the best available scientific information. However, the ways in which experts' opinions and "standard practice" evolve are complex. Variation in clinical practice, comparisons of practice with evidence-based standards, and evaluations of the recommendations of clinical experts suggest that expert opinion and "standard practice" do not provide adequate mechanisms for the transfer of scientific information into clinical decision-making.'[8]

The Bolam standard according to this view, does little to narrow the gap between established patterns of practice and evidence-based practice.[9] Dr Iain Chalmers, the Director of the UK Cochrane Centre, cites the uptake of prophylactic steroids for pregnant women likely to deliver premature babies with immature lungs as a case in point; he notes that the Royal College of Obstetricians did not officially recommend this therapy until many years after its efficacy had been scientifically established:

'Liggins and Howie first showed that antenatal corticosteroids were effective in reducing serious neonatal morbidity and mortality more than 20 years ago. Their findings were strengthened by the results of at least 13 subsequent randomised controlled trials. The strength of the evidence was made clear in a systematic review published by Crowley in 1989, and in an article and commentary published in January 1990, in the journal of the Royal College of Obstetricians and Gynaecologists. It was not until three years later, however, that the College eventually encouraged all obstetric units to "consider the use of such therapy when delivery is likely before 34 weeks".

The substantial delay between the availability of strong scientific evidence and the College's recommendation raises at least two questions. First, at which point during the past 20 years will it be judged to have been negligent not to administer steroids when there were no clear contraindications? Second, is it possible that the target of litigants will not be individual obstetricians, but the body responsible for educating them?'[10]

One aspect of Chalmers' first question has been addressed by UK law. Individual doctors *do* have a responsibility to be aware of the results of research which bear upon how they should practice. In the case of *Crawford v Board of Governors of Charing Cross Hospital*, Lord Justice Denning considered whether and when doctors were required to adopt new clinical practices in view of the explosion of published clinical reports in the 1950s. He ruled in 1953 that:

'... it would be quite wrong to suggest that the medical man is negligent because he does not at once put into operation the suggestion that some contributor or other might make in a medical journal... The time may come in a particular case when a new recommendation may be so well proved and so well known, and so well accepted that it should be adopted, but that was not so in this case.'[11]

This judgment shows that though common law does not equate scientifically validated advice with the standard of care required by law it is not blind to questions of medical effectiveness.[12] The key elements of Denning's test are:

- proof
- dissemination
- acceptance
- adoption

each in combination with the notion of wide professional approval over time. Atypical or bizarre guidelines, and 'consensus' guidelines which fail to achieve professional acceptance, would be expected to fail this test. But doctors adopting new practices advocated by guidelines based upon valid research findings issued with the aim of *hastening* incorporation of evidence-based practices into routine care are unlikely to fall foul of this test, as long as the guideline recommendations can be shown to be well proven.[7] It could be argued that 13 randomized trials and a systematic review establishing the effectiveness and safety of prophylactic steroids in the example Chalmers cites clearly meet the criteria of 'efficacy and safety tested by experience' advocated in the medical negligence text quoted above.

Chalmers also asks whether failure to adopt a practice that has *not* been widely accepted by the profession could incur liability. As things stand currently, so long as expert witnesses were prepared to testify that not giving steroids in these circumstances was a practice adopted by responsible practitioners, the courts would be likely to accept this standard of care. A Canadian health care lawyer has observed: 'the law does not require that all physicians always be at the forefront of their profession'.[2] But if it could be shown to a court's satisfaction that the omission of prophylactic steroids, though customary, constituted extreme folly (as discussed in Chapter 4), then notwithstanding its customary nature, the omission could be viewed as a breach of duty and therefore negligent.[13]

The dangers of using clinical guidelines to effect changes in customary practice is illustrated by new guidelines on the treatment of obesity, issued by the Royal College of Physicians in 1997.[14] These placed new emphasis upon the role of centrally-acting appetite-suppressants in treating obesity, countering customary practice and advice previously issued to the medical profession by the General Medical Council which stated that:

'centrally-acting appetite-suppressants, diuretics and thyroid hormones are of no real value in the treatment of obesity, as they do not benefit patients in the long term and can produce harmful side-effects.'[15]

The Royal College guidelines (prepared at the behest of the Department of Health) had to be withdrawn on the day its guidelines were further publicized by a summary article in the College's Journal.[16] A 'stop press' flyer explained to readers that new information on the safety of the treatment advocated by its guidelines had resulted in the drugs concerned being banned by the US Food and Drug Administration and withdrawn from sale in the UK.[17] Although the customary care standard suffers from the disadvantage of lagging behind evidence-based standards, it carries the advantage of its safety being more likely to have been tested by time and professional experience.

Liability of authors or sponsors

Chalmers asks whether an official organization such as a Royal College could be held liable for professional failures in the adoption of sound practice, a question also raised by the obesity guidelines episode. The answer must depend upon whether the official body concerned could be held to have a duty of care towards practitioners in the field. Generally speaking, clinical specialists are not viewed by the courts as dependent upon such bodies for their educational updating or continuous postgraduate learning. The NHSE's view on this is that:

'While an action could be taken against a clinician for not keeping up-to-date, a College is probably not actionable, as it would be difficult to show it owes a duty or obligation directly to the patient.'[18]

There are as yet no common law cases in the UK in which the courts have had to consider whether authors of clinical advice or guidelines for doctors could be liable for incorrect or misleading statements in circumstances where patients have suffered harm as a result of reliance upon them. However, in non-medical spheres, courts have been called upon to decide similar questions where individuals have claimed to have suffered economic loss by relying upon written statements. It is worth considering these cases briefly since some legal points arising from them are relevant.

The question of authors' liability for written advisory statements has arisen in the UK in cases where experts have been relied upon for advice when certain transactions are in view. These include the reports of accountants, architects, auditors and surveyors. In the case of *Candler v Crane Christmas & Co Ltd* (1951) the plaintiff invested money in a limited company relying on the accounts prepared by the company accountants, but these were found to be misleading and inaccurate. Lord Justice Denning concluded (in a dissenting judgment, but one which has since been acclaimed by the Law Lords):

'... that a duty to use care in statement is recognised by English law, and that its recognition does not create any dangerous precedent when it is remembered that it is limited in respect of the persons by whom and to whom it is owed and the transactions to which it applies.'[19]

The House of Lords has recently reviewed the law in this area. In the case of *Caparo Industries plc v Dickman and others* (1990) their Lordships made it clear that generally there can be no duty of care between the author of a document or book and its myriad potential readers, unless the authors could reasonably have foreseen that their written advice would be directly communicated to a particular reader, or class of readers, who would reasonably be expected to rely upon it.[20] They quote from an earlier judgment:

'... where a statement is put into more or less general circulation and may foreseeably be relied on by strangers... for any one of a variety of different purposes which the maker of the statement has no specific reason to anticipate... to hold the maker of the statement to be under a duty of care in respect of the accuracy of the statement to all and sundry for any purpose for which they may choose to rely on it is... to subject him, in the classic words of Cardozo CJ, to "liability in an indeterminate amount for an indeterminate time to an indeterminate class" (see *Ultramares Corp v Touche* (1931)).'[20]

The courts recognize the importance of drawing firm boundaries around the sorts of situation in which author liability may arise. In an earlier case in which the House of Lords considered these issues, it recognized, for example, that:

'A single statement may be repeated endlessly with or without the permission of its author and may be relied upon in a different way by many different people. Thus the postulate of a simple duty to avoid any harm that is with hindsight reasonably capable of being foreseen becomes untenable without the imposition of some intelligible limits to keep the law of negligence within the bounds of common sense and practicality.'[21]

The courts have therefore tried to confine possible liability to situations where a special relationship clearly exists between writer and reader. In explaining what this means the Law Lords cite a New Zealand case (*Scott Group Ltd v McFarlane* (1978)) approvingly:

'The question in any given case is whether the nature of the relationship is such that any one party can fairly be held to have assumed a responsibility to the other as regards the reliability of the advice and information. I do not think such a relationship should be found to exist unless, at least, the maker of the statement was, or ought to have been, aware that his advice or information would in fact be made available to and be relied on by a particular person or class of persons for the purposes of a particular transaction . . .'[22]

In the 1990 case of *Caparo Industries plc v Dickman and others*, Lord Oliver spelt out the nature of this special relationship after scrutiny of a previous case considered by the House of Lords, *Hedley Byrne & Co Ltd v Hellier & Partners Ltd* (1963). A special relationship of this sort can be held to exist between:

'the maker of a statement or the giver of advice (the adviser) and the recipient who acts in reliance on it (the advisee). . . where
   (1)   the advice is required for a purpose. . . which is made known, either actually or inferentially, to the adviser at the time when the advice is given
   (2)   the adviser knows either actually or inferentially, that his advice will be communicated to the advisee, either specifically or as a member of an ascertainable class, in order that it should be used by the advisee for that purpose
   (3)   it is known, either actually or inferentially, that the advice so communicated is likely to be acted on by the advisee for that purpose *without independent inquiry*
   (4)   it is so acted on by the advisee to his detriment.'[23]

In medical practice, such advisers would require to possess, and to be credited by relevant practitioners ('advisees') as possessing, quite extraordinary authority if it were to be expected that doctors should follow their advice *'without independent inquiry'*.

One difference between the legal cases considered here and the medical scenario which interests us, is that the relationship would not be a direct one between a member of the public and the authors of written advice, but between a member of the public (a patient) and an intermediary, namely the clinician who had read and acted upon advice in the form of guidelines. Traditionally, the courts expect medical professionals to act as 'learned intermediaries', interpreting the relevance of 'expert advice' in the context of each clinical problem before them. In other words, doctors are expected to exercise appropriate discretion and judgment, and not to apply advice mechanically, irrespective of relevant individual factors.

A respected health service lawyer agrees with this conclusion and reminds us that:

'the courts have been very reluctant to make one party liable for the negligent act of another person. It would be exceptional for the failure of a doctor to administer proper care to be made the responsibility of those who promoted the guideline.'[24]

Nevertheless, it has been suggested that one or two written statements of advice, such as those contained in *Martindale's Extra Pharmacopoeia* might indeed possess the status of definitive works of reference such that doctors could safely rely upon their recommendations, without independent enquiry.[25] A court case addressing this question indirectly has suggested otherwise. In the case of *Vernon v Bloomsbury Health Authority* (1995) the plaintiff, Barbara Vernon, was treated in University College Hospital in 1982 for culture negative bacterial endocarditis. She received doses of gentamycin higher than those recommended by the *Product Data Sheet*, the *British National Formulary (BNF)*, the *Monthly Index of Medical Specialities (MIMS)* and *Martindale's Extra Pharmacopoeia*, and for a period longer than that recommended by *MIMS* and *Martindale's*. She had been given 5.625 mg/kg of the drug for 19 days, whereas these reference sources at the time recommended a maximum dose of 5 mg/kg for seven days; as a consequence of this treatment she suffered bilateral vestibular damage.

At the hearing, all but one of the expert witnesses testified that they themselves would have prescribed gentamycin at this dosage for a patient in Barbara Vernon's condition. Although the plaintiff's expert witness stated that she would not herself have administered such a high dose for this condition, she was unable to say that no reasonably competent microbiologist would have prescribed at this level. The judge found that:

'... the dosage was a proper one. The doctors were not negligent in prescribing it. I agree with the defendants' experts that the guidelines laid down by the manufacturers and, for example, *MIMS*, are too conservative and that they err on the side of caution. I accept the views expressed by Dr Sowton, Dr Reeves and Dr Cooke, all of whom have great practical experience of prescribing this drug. In particular, I rely on the views of Dr Reeves. He has consistently prescribed higher doses than those recommended by the manufacturers and has advised others to do the same.'[26]

The case highlights two important points; first, that there is no expectation on the part of the courts that recommendations of medical reference works with the standing of *Martindale's Extra Pharmacopoeia* should be automatically translated into clinical practice; and second, that courts continue to place the testimony of expert witnesses concerning what constitutes reasonable practice, above that of the recommendations of prestigious works of reference. A like case, *Rodriguez v Jackson*, involving antituberculous treatment had been analysed in a very similar way by a US court in 1977.[27]

But in *Snyder v American Association of Blood Banks* (1996), a New Jersey Supreme Court found a trade association of voluntary blood banks liable to a patient for omitting to advise its member blood bank associations to institute measures that would lessen the likelihood of AIDS transmission in blood transfusions.[28] Though without precedent in the area of US medical malpractice actions, third parties responsible for safety standards in other areas of activity have been held to owe a duty of care to members of the public.[29] US courts have also held that a doctor's failure to protest against review rules in the case of a patient harmed by adherence to these rules does *not* automatically protect the review organization from liability. The case of *Wilson v Blue Cross of Southern California* (1990) involved a depressed patient who committed suicide after early discharge from hospital as a result of a decision by Blue Cross to refuse payment for any further hospital care. The court found that:

'a decision not to approve further hospitalization was a substantial factor in bringing about the decedent's demise.'[30]

In the USA, therefore, it seems likely that developers and issuers of clinical guidelines could be held liable for omitting to provide appropriate guidance, and if adherence to substandard guidelines is found to be the prime cause of patient harm.

The legal status of recommendations could generally be made clearer to doctors by emphasizing that they should *not* be adopted by clinicians 'without independent inquiry'. A recent UK collection of clinical guidelines, sent unsolicited to every general practice in the country, adopted this approach, stating:

'Readers are strongly advised to refer to the data sheets when a clinical guideline summary describes a drug therapy or when full details and the clinical significance of the products' contraindications, special precautions, drug interactions, adverse reactions or overdoses are required. While every care has been taken to ensure the accuracy of the clinical guideline summaries, this does not diminish the requirement to exercise clinical judgment and the publishers cannot accept liability for any errors and omissions.'[31]

Whilst reading like the disclaimer which it is certainly intended to be, such a statement clearly places clinical discretion at the heart of appropriate use of guidelines.

Discretion in the use of protocols and guidelines

A health lawyer has argued that tensions are bound to arise between clinical guidelines and clinical discretion:

'As clinical guidelines receive increasing acceptance in the clinical community, it may be open to argument that acting in accordance with a clinical guideline is *per se* acceptable in medical practice. The problem with this argument is that it effectively denies the importance of clinical discretion and suggests that the primary responsibility for determining the boundaries of proper medical practice rests less with the clinician than with the body formulating clinical guidelines. Unless clinical guidelines were to be elevated to the status of rules to determine appropriate clinical practice, it is highly unlikely that such an argument would succeed in an English court.'[32]

As we have seen, several legal cases exemplify how permissively the courts may interpret clinical advisory statements. The case of *Vernon v Bloomsbury Health Authority* (1995) has demonstrated the leeway a court can grant to clinicians if, despite breaching unambiguous recommendations of considerable authority, their care meets the *Bolam* standard. In the USA, deviation from clinical guidelines issued by the

American Heart Association was found to have been acceptable by a US court after unrefuted evidence that:

'. . . the American Heart Association's guidelines are mere guidelines that may be altered by the physician.'[33]

Courts in the UK have no fixed view about the obligations (if any) which guidelines may express about how doctors should behave in particular situations. In the case of *Ratty v Haringey Health Authority and another* (1994), a surgeon was exonerated from a charge of negligence by the Court of Appeal after the Court accepted that 'Marnham's Rule', which asserts that abdomino-perineal resection should only be performed where there is histological proof of malignancy, should be viewed only as 'a useful guideline... not one to be followed in every case'.[34] On the other hand, in the case of *Wilsher v Essex Area Health Authority* (1986), which involved an action brought by a premature baby who suffered blindness after prolonged oxygen-enriched ventilation, the plaintiff's expert witness would not agree with defence counsel that the safe upper limit for a baby's arterial pO_2 could be described as 'merely a guideline', as severe risk to the baby's eyesight supervened above this level.[35]

The NHSE stated in 1996 that even when endorsed by prestigious professional bodies:

'or commended by the NHS Executive, clinical guidelines can still only assist the practitioner; they cannot be used to mandate, authorise or outlaw treatment options. Regardless of the strength of the evidence, it will remain the responsibility of the practising clinicians to interpret their application taking account of local circumstances and the needs and wishes of individual patients. It would be wholly inappropriate for clinical guidelines to be used as a means of coercion of the individual clinician, by managers and senior professionals.'[18]

Rigid uncritical adherence to guidelines is neither a legal, nor according to official pronouncements, the managerial expectation. Even where a guideline has been laid down as a legal standard, its appropriate application may still require the exercise of discretion. In the case of *McFarlane v Secretary of State for Scotland* (1988), Mr McFarlane appealed to the Sheriff Court in Scotland, against a decision by the Secretary of State to revoke his driving licence after uncontested findings that his field of vision did not amount to the minimum recommended by the Royal College of Ophthalmologists, at least 20 degrees above and below the horizontal.[36]

Expert testimony centred on the congenital nature of the appellant's defect, which was neither degenerative nor progressive, and to which he had fully adapted. McFarlane suffered from a left upper homonymous quadrantanopia which it was deemed would have little significance to a driver looking straight ahead, or from side to side in the rear mirror. The Sheriff noted that the Secretary of State's advisers had 'simply followed the recommendations in the guidelines laid down'.[36] The court found that Mr McFarlane was not a danger to the public and his driving licence was duly reinstated.

The case highlights the importance of appreciating that advisory statements should probably never be thought of as hard and fast rules, but always require to be interpreted by a proper exercise of discretion.[37] Administrative law generally allows decision-makers:

'... to develop and apply flexible guidelines to structure the exercise of their discretionary powers, provided they are not used rigidly so as to exclude the essence of discretion, namely a readiness to deal with each case on its merits.'

In administrative law terms, the essence of discretion is choice, but as a leading textbook notes, discretion may be:

'... limited, without being entirely removed, by standards or guidelines or criteria which the decision-maker is to take into account in exercising discretion.'[38]

Some clinical guidelines, such as those issued by the World Health Organization for the treatment of hypertension,[39] explicitly recognize that translating precepts into action requires discretion, just as the exercise of discretion frequently involves using rules sensibly:[40]

'Guidelines should provide extensive, critical, and well balanced information on benefits and limitations of the various diagnostic and therapeutic interventions so that the physician may exert the most careful judgment in individual cases.'[39]

The role of clinical discretion being advocated here can usefully be likened to its central importance when prescribing licensed medicines for unlicensed clinical indications. The licensing of a medicine for certain indications provides a limited guarantee of quality, safety and efficacy in specified clinical situations, but doctors in the UK are not obliged by law to prescribe only within such indications. As a recent reviewer observed:

'Doctors have traditionally exercised their clinical freedom in prescribing drugs for unlicensed indications for the patient's benefit. However, if they decide to go beyond the limits set out in the licence they should only do so after careful thought.'[41]

The position can be further complicated where official guidelines advise doctors to use drugs for unlicensed indications, such as the 1997 *Guidelines for the Prevention of Malaria in Travellers from the United Kingdom*. These guidelines recommend doxycycline be used for the prophylaxis of falciparum malaria in people travelling to certain parts of the world even though doxycycline is not licensed for this indication. Issued by the Public Health Laboratory Service's Communicable Diseases Surveillance Centre, the guidelines contain a full statement of the working methods of the development group, but state that:

'The views expressed in these guidelines reflect experienced professional opinion, since the data are inadequate for unequivocal views to be given on several issues. There is often a range of acceptable options... Decisions on the terms under which different drugs are licensed for use are the responsibility of the Licensing Authority... (not of these guidelines). The guidelines should be read as a supplement to and not as a substitute for the relevant data sheets.'[42]

Tensions have surfaced in US courts between the clinical judgment of physicians and the treatment protocols they have followed, but doctors have been unable to pass off liability for injuries caused to patients by claiming that they were merely following official guidance or guidelines. In the case of *Wickline v State of California* (1986), the court decided that a doctor could not claim as a defence to negligence, that his or her clinical judgment had been corrupted by clinical guidelines:

'[A] physician who complies without protest... when his medical judgment dictates otherwise, cannot avoid responsibility for his patient's care.'[43]

The case involved early discharge of a patient according to a 'Medi-Cal utilization review protocol' consisting of treatment guidelines, including length of stay criteria approved for payment purposes. As a result of too early a discharge, it was alleged that the patient had to undergo an amputation, and that the physician who had allowed the discharge to take place had thereby been negligent. The doctor had not protested against the Medi-Cal guidelines because he believed a request for extended hospitalization would have been refused. Expert testimony stated that the doctor's decision to allow discharge, at the time when he did, fell within the boundaries of the customary standard of care. He was therefore not found liable in negligence. However, the court held that there was an obligation upon a physician, in circumstances where a patient's condition could benefit from further hospitalization, to appeal for an extension of hospital stay, even if such extension was likely to have been refused. Appropriate attention to non-directive terminology, and avoidance by guideline developers of terms such as 'never' and 'always' will help ensure that doctors appreciate that guideline use is no substitute for appropriate clinical judgment.[44]

Chapters 3, 4 and 5 have outlined how clinical guidelines interact and intersect with the law in different ways. Legislation has both alighted upon, and been influential in developing, the regulatory effects of clinical guidelines. Common law cases, however, have not yet credited guidelines with any special 'self-evident' status as regards the legal value of the standards they embody. Courts have not followed standards taken from guidelines without critically evaluating their authority, applicability and flexibility and most crucially of all, the extent to which they represent customary practice.

That guidelines have not been pivotal in influencing court outcome is a conclusion supported by the only large scale study that has investigated this question. Undertaken in the USA, this study found that guidelines had 'a relevant or pivotal role in the proof of negligence' in only 6.6% of medical malpractice actions.[45]

These findings should reassure doctors who harbour fears that guideline proliferation increases the risk of being found liable in negligence actions. Whether guidelines are likely to erode clinical judgment, to reduce medical practice to a series of mechanistic rule-following activities, and whether guidelines threaten clinical freedom, are questions considered in the final chapter.

Summary

The Bolam test of the standard of clinical care required by law appears to hinder attempts to narrow differences between customary patterns of medical practice and evidence-based practice.

Though the law is not blind to questions of medical effectiveness, common law does not automatically equate scientifically validated medical treatment with the legally required standard of care.

The customary care Bolam standard suffers from the possible disadvantage of lagging behind evidence-based standards, but may carry the advantage of its safety having been tested by time and wide professional experience.

Clinical guidelines designed to hasten the incorporation of evidence-based practices into routine care must be well validated in risk/benefit terms to patients, especially if the guidelines advocate treatment patterns that significantly depart from customary care.

In the UK, it is unlikely that authors or sponsors of faulty guidelines will be held liable for patient injury, because the courts expect the treating clinician always to exercise appropriate discretion and judgment and not to apply advice mechanically.

The legal status of recommendations contained in guidelines should be made clearer to doctors.

References

1 Bolitho v City & Hackney Health Authority (1997) 3 *WLR*: 1151–61.
2 Jutras D (1993) Clinical practice guidelines as practice norms. *Can Med Assoc J*. **148**: 905–8.
3 Robins AW and Lloyd BW (1995) Most consultants deviate from asthma guidelines. [Letter]. *BMJ*. **311**: 508.
4 British Asthma Guidelines Coordinating Committee (1997) British guidelines on asthma management: 1995 review and position statement. *Thorax*. **52**: S1–24.
5 Nathan PC and Barrowclough AR (1957) *Medical Negligence*. Butterworths, London, p. 28.
6 Landau v Werner (1961) **105** *Sol Jo*: 1008 (CA). Quoted in Kennedy I and Grubb A (1994) *Medical Law: text and materials*. Second ed. Butterworths, London, p. 1073.
7 Haines A and Jones R (1994) Implementing findings of research. *BMJ*. **308**: 1488–92.
8 Oxman AD, Sackett MD and Guyatt GH (1993) Users' guides to the medical literature. *JAMA*. **270**: 2093.

9   Chalmers I (1994) Why are opinions about the effects of health care so often wrong? *Medico-Legal Journal.* 62/3: 116–30. Transcript of a talk given to the Medico-Legal Society in November 1993 by the Director of the UK Cochrane Centre.

10   Chalmers I (1993) Underuse of antenatal corticosteroids and future litigation. [Letter]. *Lancet.* 341: 699.

11   Crawford v Board of Governors of Charing Cross Hospital (1953) In: Mason J and McCall Smith R (eds) (1991) *Law and Medical Ethics.* Butterworths, London, p. 211.

12   Schyve PM (1993) Judges as gatekeepers: guidelines in court. *J Qual Improvement.* 19: 283–90.

13   Holyoak J (1990) Raising the standard of medical care. *Legal Studies.* 10: 201–11.

14   Royal College of Physicians (1997) *Overweight and Obese Patients: principles of management with particular reference to the use of drugs.* RCP, London.

15   General Medical Council (1993) *News Review.* GMC, London, 3: 2.

16   Jung R (1997) Managing overweight and obese patients with particular reference to the use of drugs. *J Roy Coll Phys Lond.* 31: 506–8.

17   Royal College of Physicians (1997) *Stop Press Statement: Withdrawal of recommendations. Overweight and Obese Patients: principles of management with particular reference to the use of drugs.* RCP, London, 15 September.

18   NHS Executive (1996) *Clinical Guidelines: using clinical guidelines to improve patient care within the NHS.* DoH, London, p. 10.

19   Candler v Crane Christmas & Co Ltd (1951) 1 *All ER*: 426–50 at 436.

20   Caparo Industries plc v Dickman and others (1990) 1 *All ER*: 568–608.

21   Hedley Byrne & Co Ltd v Hellier & Partners Ltd (1963) 2 *All ER*: 575–618.

22   Scott Group Ltd v McFarlane (1978) 1 *New Zealand LR*: 553.

23   Caparo Industries plc v Dickman and others (1990) 1 *All ER*: 568–608 at 589.

24   Newdick C (1995) *Who Should We Treat?* Clarendon Press, Oxford, p. 178.

25   Brahams D and Wyatt J (1989) Decision aids and the law. *Lancet.* ii: 632–4.

26   Vernon v Bloomsbury Health Authority (1995) 6 *Med LR*: 297–310.

27   Rodriguez v Jackson (1977) 574 *Pacific Reporter 2d Series*: 481–6.

28 Snyder v American Association of Blood Banks (1996) **676** *Atlantic Reporter 2d Series*: 1036–64.

29 Noble A, Brennan T and Hyams A (1998) Snyder v American Association of Blood Banks: a re-examination of liability for medical practice guideline promulgators. *J Evaluation in Clinical Practice*. In press.

30 Wilson v Blue Cross of Southern California (1990) **271** *Cal Rptr 3rd Series*: 876–85.

31 Anonymous (1997) *Guidelines – summarising clinical guidelines for primary care*. Mebendium, Berkhamsted. **1**: 4.

32 Stern K (1995) Clinical guidelines and negligence liability. In: Deighan M and Hitch S (eds) *Clinical Effectiveness: from guidelines to cost-effective practice*. Earlybrave Publications Ltd, Brentwood, pp. 127–35.

33 Lowry v Henry Mayo Newhall Memorial Hospital (CA) (1990) **229** *Cal Rptr*: 620.

34 Ratty v Haringey Health Authority and another (1993) (Court of Appeal Civil Division). *Lexis Manuscript*. Mead Data Central, OH.

35 Wilsher v Essex Area Health Authority (1986) **3** *All ER*: 801–36.

36 McFarlane v Secretary of State for Scotland (1988) *Scottish Civil LR*: 623–8.

37 Hurwitz B (1994) Clinical guidelines: proliferation and medico-legal significance. *Quality in Health Care*. **3**: 37–44.

38 Cane P (1992) *An Introduction to Administrative Law*. Clarendon Press, Oxford, p. 132.

39 Subcommittee of ISH/World Health Organisation Mild Hypertension Liaison Committee (1993) Summary of 1993 WHO International Society of Hypertension guidelines for the management of mild hypertension. *BMJ*. **307**: 1541–6.

40 Hawkins K (1992) The use of legal discretion: perspectives from law and social science. In: Hawkins K (ed.) *The Uses of Discretion*. Clarendon Press, Oxford, pp. 11–46.

41 Ferner RE (1996) Prescribing licensed medicines for unlicensed indications. *Prescribers' J*. **36**: 73–8.

42 Bradley DJ and Warhurst DC (on behalf of an expert group of doctors, nurses and pharmacists) (1997) *Guidelines for the Prevention of Malaria in Travellers from the United Kingdom*. Centre for Communicable Diseases, London.

43 Wickline v State of California (1986) **228** *Cal Rptr*: 661, 667.

44 Spernak SM, Budetti PP and Zweig F (1992) *Use of Language in Clinical Practice Guidelines*. Centre for Health Policy Research,

Agency for Health Care Policy and Research, Rockville, MD, pp. 1–16.

45 Hyams AL, Brandenburg JA, Lipsitz SR *et al.* (1995) Practice guidelines and malpractice litigation: a two-way street. *Ann Intrn Med.* **122**: 450–5.

6 Guidelines, Clinical Judgment and Clinical Freedom

In their clinical work doctors synthesize generalizable knowledge and practical skills with specific knowledge of, and concern for, particular patients. The philosopher Stephen Toulmin once observed that from classical times onwards, clinical medicine has presented thinkers with intriguing examples of the 'close alliance of mind and hand, theory and practice, universal and existential'.[1] How do clinical guidelines fit into these processes, and if they do, what challenges do they pose to clinical practice as we know it?

Consideration of some of these matters is of longstanding. In the 3rd century BC, the philosopher Plato explored the difference between skills grounded in practical expertise, and those based merely upon following instruction or obeying rules. Using the clinician as his model, Plato set up a thought-experiment: doctors would be stripped of their clinical freedom – 'no longer allowed unchecked authority' – but form themselves into councils which would then dictate the majority view of how to practise medicine in all situations.[2]

'Visitor: ... suppose... that we were to make it a matter of policy that members of the... profession are no longer allowed unchecked authority over anyone... We decide to convene ourselves into an assembly... We make it possible for anyone to voice an opinion about sickness, whether or not he has any professional knowledge... He can suggest how we are to use drugs and medical equipment in treating the sick...

Once the assembly has heard all this advice, whether it has come from doctors... or else from laymen, the majority decision about these matters is written up on the official notice-boards and inscribed on stelae... and from then on it dictates the ways in which the treatment of the sick is practised.

Young Socrates: You've certainly thought up a strange scenario.

Visitor: Anyone who wants to can prosecute any of the rulers for having failed... to direct... our written code... for healing the sick... So, Socrates, suppose this scenario of ours really happened. What would the effect be?

Young Socrates: Obviously, it would completely obliterate expertise in all its forms...'[2]

Plato's notion of codifying the majority decisions of panels (composed of clinical and non-clinical members), and official publication of the results in order to influence (Plato says *to dictate*) 'the ways in which the treatment of the sick is practised' prefigures, in a remarkable way, many of the impulses which animate the clinical guidelines movement in the present day.[3]

In Plato's view, important hallmarks of expertise include flexible responsiveness and 'improvisatory ability' – an approach to practice endangered, he believed, by use of guidelines.[2,4] However effective health care by guideline turned out to be – and Plato seemed prepared to concede its potential – it remained in his view a debased form of practice, because guidelines presuppose an 'average patient' rather than a *particular* patient whom the doctor treats, and because the knowledge and analysis that go into the creation of guidelines are not rooted in the mental processes of clinicians but in the minds of guideline developers distant from the consultation.

Once the profession has committed itself to providing health care through guidelines, Plato saw no alternative but to ensure compliance with them, even if this entailed resorting to legal action. Such guidelines had to be considered to be treated as 'clinical laws'. For once expertise resides no longer within the patient's clinician but is represented in guidelines instead, corruption of or deviation from them would result in treatment based merely upon personal whim or quackery:

'Visitor: Suppose... we elected an official to supervise the regulations, but he didn't care about them in the slightest and set about infringing them, not because he knew what he was doing, but because he'd been bribed, or because he owed someone a personal favour. This would be an even worse state of affairs, wouldn't it, though the previous scenario was bad enough?

Young Socrates: You're quite right.

Visitor: Yes, he'd be infringing the results of a great deal of experience, I think, and a great deal of clever advice and persuasive argument. That's what it took for the laws to become established, and to go about infringing them would be to commit a far worse error and would undermine all kinds of activities far more effectively than a written legal code.

Young Socrates:　Of course it would.

Visitor:　And that is why, when laws and statutes *have* been established (whatever situation they may apply to), the second-best course is to prevent any individual or any body of people from ever infringing them in the slightest.'[2]

In Plato's understanding, expertise is founded upon systematic knowledge and clinical experience grounded in the mental processes of physicians exercising clinical judgment. It depends not only upon the possession of knowledge, but crucially, upon its effective application. Plato returned to the possible deleterious effects of guidelines upon medical practice in another dialogue. Here, he termed doctors who were slaves or cared for slaves, and who learn their trade merely by imitation, 'doctors' assistants':

'Athenian:　... with doctors, you know, when we're ill: one follows one method of treatment, one another... we usually speak, I think, of doctors and doctors' assistants, but of course we call the latter 'doctors' too... And these 'doctors' (who may be free men or slaves) pick up the skill empirically, by watching and obeying their masters; they've no systematic knowledge such as the free doctors have learned for themselves and pass on to their pupils.

Athenian:　... It wasn't a bad parallel we made, you know, when we compared all those for whom legislation is produced today to slaves under treatment from slave doctors. Make no mistake about what would happen, if one of those doctors who are innocent of theory and practise medicine by rule of thumb were ever to come across a gentleman doctor conversing with a gentleman patient. This doctor would be acting almost like a philosopher, engaging in a discussion that ranged over the source of the disease and pushed the enquiry back into the whole nature of the body.'[5]

For Plato, the effectiveness which guideline use could confer was predicated upon very low levels of understanding on the part of user clinicians. He foresaw that imposition of guidelines upon an educated medical profession would threaten the intellectual autonomy of the profession, and result in poorer clinical care in the long run.

Clinical judgment

In these dialogues, Plato adeptly alighted upon issues which continue to trouble clinicians to this day; concerning the rationality of medical practice, the nature of clinical judgment, and the role of an active and enquiring mind in medical practice. In the 20th century, doctors remain fearful that widespread use of guidelines could erode clinical abilities, inhibit judgment, and reduce clinical practice to thoughtless activities performed by physician automata.[6,7]

Plato conceptualized guidelines as socially engineered rules governing medical decisions; clinical decision-making would thereby move from the private realm of the doctor–patient relationship, into a public realm permitting scrutiny and review of clinical decisions using guidelines as criteria. But can such rules ever be completely and properly formulated to cover the myriad of potential clinical situations with which doctors are daily confronted? Modern day philosophers have pointed out that just because a treatment is likely to offer benefits does not mean that, all things considered, it should be administered:

'The medical judgment that [treatment] is indicated does not entail the ethical judgment that it ought to be administered to a particular patient... Judgments of medical indication do not command the patient [or doctor] categorically but give medical advice.'[8]

Patients may wish to take risks and to avoid certain adverse effects of treatments. Opinionated judgments on the part of doctors, grounded in clinical experience, counterweighted by knowledge of scientific findings, and sensitive to patients' wishes are not simple transductions of 'input information' which result in 'output decisions'.[9,10] Even where doctor and patient *agree* on the desirability of a treatment, when and how it is introduced, the pace at which dosages may be altered and with what tolerability by the individual patient, are only a few of the many factors likely to be considered in decision-making processes. Clinical judgments go beyond explicit input information, adding considerations of feeling, attitude, and value to the output.[10] Such judgments concern complex individual circumstances, and are frequently undertaken in the context of different degrees of uncertainty, where opinions may differ, and where the authority of sense perceptions and intuitions can play inter-active roles.

Cognitive psychologists have identified many processes at work in clinical decision-making, including apprehension and discernment of alternative courses of action. Once different options have been character-ized and their likely consequences understood, the doctor, in dialogue with the patient, chooses the most appropriate course in the light of the circumstances, bearing in mind the patient's wishes. Though to varying degrees the judgments required of clinicians in discrete areas of medicine, such as diagnosis or the management of chronic conditions, can be successfully specified, this does not *reduce* clinical judgment to nothing other than 'decisional algebra' that can be objectified in expert systems, algorithms, and guidelines.

Selection, estimation and classification play their part in clinical judg-ment which should not be viewed as a unitary process. The American physician, Alvan Feinstein, draws particular attention to the intermingling of formal and informal knowledge, with subjective and objective considerations frequently required during clinical decision-making:

'The physician knows the many clinical distinctions that tell him when death is imminent or hope abundant; when to treat and when to wait; when to sedate with drugs and when to sedate with words; when to stop treatment, change or add; when to treat aggressively for cure, palliatively for relief and consolingly for comfort. The physician knows that these therapeutic decisions may depend on such distinctively bedside observations as the strength of the patient's handgrip, the posture of his body, the noise in his chest, the smell of his breath, the sweat of his brow, the grimace on his face, the quiver in his voice and the anguish of his family. The physician knows that the therapeutic decision may depend on such distinctly clinical nuances as a particular continuation of symptoms and signs, whether the patient complains of certain symptoms or tolerates them quietly, whether the disease was found before or after the symptoms developed, whether the symptoms were of short duration or long, and whether the symptoms had prece-ded one another or followed. The good clinician knows all these things and many more distinctly clinical features that are his harbingers of prognosis and determinants of therapy. But he cannot express these specifically or consistently.'[11]

Clinical judgments are often extended over time, and call upon complex skills requiring intimate understanding of how biological processes intersect with personal biographical ones. These dialogic and narrative aspects of clinical work can become obscured by attempts to construe the rationality of judgment solely in terms of a 'deductive logic' with a 'latent algorithmic form'.[12] An American physician has complained about what he terms:

'The development of a form of mathematical terrorism: clinical judgment, even if based on years of experience, knowledge of relevant studies in the medical literature, and the opinions of world experts (usually based on data from more patients with a similar problem than any of us will ever encounter), is rebuked in deference to construction of a quantitative decision analysis. When faced with a patient who has complex medical problems... I will continue to use my "clinical judgment", which is not a dirty word.'[13]

In reality, the balance between objective and subjective considerations in clinical decisions differs depending upon the nature of the patient's condition, the stage of illness reached, and the extent to which the patient wishes to be an active participant in decisions. Human sensitivity, perception and interpretation all have important roles to play in a process which utilizes skills ranging from logical analysis to intuition. A century ago, the Viennese surgeon, Wilhelm Billroth, whilst celebrating the growth of scientific medicine could also foresee its clinical limitations:

'To render medical ability independent from personal tradition, to establish the art of medicine for all time so firmly in writing that it will be independent from the talent of individuals, and to transform it wholly into a science is the ideal goal of our efforts... I doubt that this goal will ever be reached: it will at least not be reached by the art of medicine any sooner than the art of poetry dissolves into metrics, painting into colour theory or music into harmony.'[14]

It is therefore not surprising that researchers, health service managers and those involved in audit have repeatedly reported wide variations in health care practices that cannot easily be accounted for by differences in patient case-mix, or the circumstances of practice. Modern studies of decision-making confirm it to involve multiple assessments of, and interactions between, scientific evidence, patient desire, doctor preferences and 'all sorts of exogenous influences, some of which may be quite irrelevant'.[15] Indeed, one American legal scholar has observed that:

'The claim that clinical decisions are dictated by science and never by habit or folklore or economic self-interest has served the profession well in maintaining its authority and in building ideological resistance to any development threatening that authority.'[16]

Clinical guidelines have an important role to play in influencing medical decision-making in situations where there is *both* considerable certainty about efficacious treatment (based upon scientific evidence or expert opinion) *and* where significant departure from such practice occurs with no valid justification. Whilst accepting that variation in clinical practice may be justifiable because of scientific uncertainty and differences in values, the US Institute of Medicine rightly asserts variability to be unacceptable when it:

'stems from poor practitioner skills, poor management of delivery systems, ignorance, or deliberate disregard of well-documented preferable practices. It should not be tolerated when it is a self-serving disguise for bad practices that harm people and waste resources.'[17]

Compliance with valid accepted guidelines in these circumstances is likely to narrow variability in clinical practice, improve the standard of health care and provide a guarantor to patients and purchasers against the effects of bad doctoring. It is a mistake, however, to turn this argument round, to maintain that clinical guidelines are required in order to remedy wide variations, without first studying *why* such variations exist. Inherent uncertainties, lack of evidence, poor consensus, differences in patient choice and expectation, as well as legitimate clinical discretion can all contribute to differences in practice.[18]

Klim McPherson, Professor of Public Health at the University of London, has observed that legitimate variation in medical practices may not have been sufficiently appreciated by UK health service managers or purchasers keen to control costs by standardizing procedures and narrowing unit costs:[19]

'The most enthusiastic advocates for the purchasing of guidelines and protocols may have paid insufficient attention to the uncertainty 'inherent in clinical practice, with the imposition of a spurious rationality on a sometimes inherently irrational process... Most decisions are affected by many different factors, including characteristics of the doctor and the patient and their interaction... Guidelines should... only ever be used as guidelines. Purchasers seeking to convert them into restrictive protocols in contracts will have much to do to incorporate patient choice in a way that is distinguishable from the unjustifiable variation in clinical practice which they seek to combat.'[19]

Though purchasers have been urged no longer to buy treatments but treatment protocols,[20] these third party health care agencies must understand that rigid, uncritical adherence to clinical guidelines cannot be a formal, managerial or legal expectation in the NHS (as discussed in Chapter 4), and may lead to inappropriate clinical care.

Clinical freedom

In reconsidering the obituary he wrote for clinical freedom 15 years ago,[21] Professor John Hampton, has recently discussed the subject in the light of the growing importance of evidence-based medicine:

'When a patient fits neatly into a disease category covered by a trial, the results of the trial can be applied and can be supervised by a general practitioner, a nurse or indeed a computer. There are, however, many patients who do not fit neatly into the inclusion and exclusion criteria of the published trials, and many more who have complications of their disease or treatment for whom there can never be proper trial evidence on which to base management. In all such patients the doctor has to do the best he can, and needs the freedom to treat the patient as an individual in whatever seems the best way.'[22]

For doctors in Professor Hampton's situation, following the advice of rigorously developed guidelines offers both advantages and disadvantages. Since the guideline development group should have reviewed all accessible evidence bearing upon clinical management, there is less likelihood that one particular trial, perhaps the most recently published or the only one a clinician can remember, will come to dominate clinical decisions. But disadvantages stem from doubts about guideline development techniques, for example the validity of meta-analysis,[23] or the manner in which consensus has been reached, or the effect of presupposing an average patient in drawing up recommendations, rather than the particular patient whom a doctor is treating.

Graphic and personal examples of the difficulties doctors face in applying evidence-based data to individual treatment decisions were given to the 1995 House of Lords' Select Committee on Science and Technology, in which the Director of the UK Cochrane Centre, Dr Iain Chalmers said:

'Well, the evidence says this. What the *implications* of the evidence are for practice requires a judgment. For example, ... there is very clear evidence that giving oxytocic drugs, uterus contracting drugs, at the third stage [of labour] reduces post-partum haemorrhage. That does not necessarily mean that these drugs should be given routinely. If the circumstances are such that you can deal with a post-partum haemorrhage promptly, then you may decide that it is not worth giving the drug routinely. I think one has to distinguish between what the evidence says and what the evidence means.

If I was having transient ischaemic attacks I would have no doubt that – on the basis of the evidence available to me – I would want to take low dose aspirin. But I am not going to start taking low dose aspirin now because, as a result of a recent brush with the health services, I know that I am at low risk of cardiovascular complications. Although I might reduce a very low absolute risk fractionally by going on low dose aspirin, it would not, in my view, be worth my while taking the drug... that is why I say that the evidence is essential, but that it is not sufficient for coming to informed decisions.'[24]

We should therefore be careful not to constrain flexible clinical responsiveness with an approach to guideline implementation which overvalues the scientific base. Such an approach would result in a pseudoscientific clinical discipline, aptly characterized by Professor Grimley Evans:

'There is a fear that in the absence of evidence clearly applicable to the case in hand a clinician might be forced by guidelines to make use of evidence which is only doubtfully relevant, generated perhaps in a different grouping of patients in another country and some other time and using a similar but not identical treatment. This is evidence-*biased* medicine; it is to use evidence in the manner of the fabled drunkard who searched under the street lamp for his door key because that is where the light was, even though he had dropped the key somewhere else.'[25]

Accepting Klim McPherson's view that 'clinical medicine is not an exact science, and in many respects it is not a science at all, only science based',[19] can help to prevent us from expecting that, by following clinical guidelines, doctors can bypass the need to engage in the intellectually and emotionally demanding processes of making clinical judgments.[26]

Until relatively recently in historical terms, variability between doctors in their clinical judgments was viewed as a natural expression of the differing personal doctoring qualities of clinicians. Had not Hippocrates said:

'... as in all the other arts, those who practise them differ much one from another in dexterity and knowledge, so it is in like manner with Medicine?'[27]

Even 20th century physicians have celebrated the subjective aspects of clinical practice. Writing in the 1940s, the Regius Professor of Physic at

Cambridge referred to the much valued ability – some would say the *duty*[22] – of health care professionals, to exercise their clinical judgment freely, flexibly and unimpeded by external constraints:

'One of the attractions of the profession is the personal and individual character of its practice: the latitude with which a qualified doctor may exercise his own judgment, express his own opinions and practise his own art... If the profession of medicine be robbed of its scope for individuality the soul will go out of it.'[28]

On this view of medical practice, the proliferation of clinical guidelines appears to be part of a concerted strategy to 'micro-manage' the doctor–patient relationship using a system of 'cerebral constraints' which operate upon clinical decision-making, threatening the right of doctors to perform clinical work unimpeded.[29,30]

Though increasing societal regulation of health care has necessarily followed its public financing in the UK, the establishment of official complaints procedures, a health ombudsman, the GMC's performance review powers, and a vast increase in the incidence of medical negligence claims have all made inroads upon a freedom which was formerly professionally defined and professionally patrolled. In the USA, guidelines have been explicitly identified with attempts to interfere with doctors' work; in 1971, a United States appeal judge was outspoken in his condemnation of them on these grounds. In a case involving a patient who had been refused sterilization because she had not come within the clinical indication guidelines adopted by the hospital for this procedure, the judge rebuked the hospital authority in the following terms:

'Fortunately for our society, the State has wisely not undertaken to establish medical guidelines and procedures for doctors and surgeons in public hospitals. Of all professions in which the exercise of judgment should be as uncontrolled as possible, it is the medical profession.'[31]

Yet within some ten years of his judgment, Congress established Peer Review Organizations to institute review criteria for Medicare treatment programmes in an effort to control the cost of federally-funded health care (*see* Chapter 3). Despite the withdrawal of funds later allocated to the guidelines programme of the Agency for Health Care Policy and Research, guideline imposed care has probably attained its most developed and pervasive form within 'managed care' programmes in the USA. One commentator has written that:

'In managed care's arsenal of cost-control weaponry, probably none is more potent – except restricting hospital admission – than superseding the physician's autonomy by a managerial-review process in which armies of claim clerks, administrators, and technocrats of every description insinuate themselves into a complex system that authorizes, delivers, and pays for medical services.'[32]

There seems little doubt that the harsh effects of restraining medical costs, mediated by payer-influenced clinical guidelines also threatens clinical freedom in the UK. In a book co-authored by a moral philosopher and a doctor addressing the education of clinicians, Downie and Charlton define clinical freedom as 'the freedom of a doctor to investigate, prescribe, or carry out a procedure, refer, or communicate, regardless of cost, other professional opinion, or patients', or social views, in the best interests of patients'.[33]

This definition makes clear that the moral licence to practise should not be based upon the professional licence alone, but requires to be subjected to a best interests test as well, a matter open to external review by health service management, special audits and even by the courts. Leaving aside the problem of cost, which is now testing this formulation to its limits, Downie and Charlton's definition signals the demise of a notion of clinical freedom that was both professionally defined and professionally regulated.

Best interests, however, as we have seen in Chapters 4 and 5, is not the test which underpins the standard of medical care required by law except in the case of medical treatment provided to young children, and people who are legally incompetent.[34] In the case of competent adults, UK law requires medical treatment to conform with that judged acceptable by a responsible body of practitioners, the Bolam test.[35] It can be seen, therefore, that UK common law has preserved an aspect of professionally defined and professionally countenanced clinical freedom in the test it continues to adopt in deciding upon actions alleging medical negligence.

Clinical freedom remains critical to the practice of good medicine, as Plato clearly understood. Autonomous clinical thought, which Downie and Charlton understand to be the medical profession's 'freedom to think... freedom for initiative and individual responsibility',[33] would be undermined by unthinking conformity to clinical guidelines.[36] For this reason, guideline developers should give more thought to their own expectations as to how guidelines are to be used within clinical settings; to how guideline, doctor and patient are to interact during the consultation.

Plato was right to reject a relationship that conceptualized guidelines as rules, and doctors as ruled; a partnership between guideline and user is to be preferred. For this relationship to be realized, studies must be undertaken of the cognitive processes involved in using guidelines actively and interactively, of the discretion exercised in their use, and how this differs from the discretion presupposed by other decision aids such as textbooks, lecture notes or expert computer systems. Much greater dialogue between guideline developers, guideline users, and patients must be created.

A Canadian professor of health services research, Jonathan Lomas, has argued that modern processes of guideline development and implementation have much to learn from equivalent processes in the realm of public policy legislation. Hitherto, guideline development has generally been accomplished informally, by relatively uncodified processes unavailable to public view and debate. Public policies, by contrast, are more likely to be developed by procedures accessible to public scrutiny, through formal consultation and debate.[37] The emergence of more formal guideline development techniques, outlined in Chapter 2, has gone some way towards meeting Lomas's criticisms. Unlike the consensus guidelines of Plato, modern day evidence-linked clinical guidelines seek to make transparent the strengths, weaknesses and relevance of research findings to clinical care. Even if such guidelines are sometimes formulated as behavioural rules, their appropriate interpretation and application are likely to lead to better clinical care and a safer medico-legal strategy, than either uncritical disregard or unthinking compliance.[38]

Conclusion

There is little doubt that guidelines are set to become increasingly influential in both the way doctors practise *and* the manner in which they are to be held accountable. Although there may be no official managerial requirement that doctors should automatically follow clinical guidelines (other than where they have a statutory backing), the climate and framework in which health care is provided increasingly emphasizes the value of standardized treatments promoted by guidelines.

In the 1950s, Ernest Nagel, a philosopher of science addressing issues raised by the growth of robotic automation, dismissed fears that automatic controls in the home and at work would 'deprive us of all that gives zest and value to our lives'. He believed that 'the history of science exhibits a steady tendency to eliminate intellectual effort in the solution of individualized problems, by developing comprehensive formulas which can resolve by rote a whole class of them.' Acts of thought, he contended, are mostly required 'at the critical junction of affairs'.[39]

This book has argued that such 'critical junctions' tend to arise frequently in clinical practice precisely because medicine involves evaluating the complex circumstances of individual patients who require individualized solutions to their problems and predicaments. Following comprehensive formulas of clinical management will no doubt release doctors from tedious and predictable routines but, if performed 'by rote', risks inappropriate application and depersonalization of doctor–patient and patient–doctor relationships. Neither patients nor doctors are likely to find treatments administered in this way satisfactory.

On the other hand, we have seen that developments in the extraction, digestion and the interpretation of data from medical research, together with a renewed determination to disseminate the results of these findings to practising clinicians, mean that the clinical freedom to pursue practices which fly in the face of scientifically established clinical effectiveness cannot be defended. The Bolam test is coming under pressure in the legal arena for tending to assume that the medical profession's customary practices generally constitute the legally required minimum standard of care.[40] There are also concerns that the courts are too easily influenced by expert witnesses who may not be up-to-date, and may not provide adequate reflections of customary practice,[41] though Lord Woolf's proposals to reform the procedural basis of medical negligence litigation are likely to expose expert opinions to much greater scrutiny (*see* page 42).[42,43]

Rigorously developed guidelines and protocols offer courts examples of validated clinical standards across an increasingly wide range of medical practice; as they continue to proliferate, so will they undoubtedly come to be cited in court. And there seems little doubt that courts will take note of the standards which these clinical guidelines advocate. But courts are unlikely to follow such standards slavishly, without critically appraising their authority, flexibility, scope of application, and the extent to which guidelines reflect customary responsible practice.

Despite stirrings afoot to replace the customary care standard of *Bolam* with a standard determined without any reference to customary practice, it is unlikely that guidelines will become such a standard. Legal cases reveal that clinical guidelines have not been credited by the courts with any special 'self-evident' status, and have played a subservient role to that of the expert witness in court proceedings.

Despite the claim that whoever controls clinical guidelines controls medicine itself,[44] the common law looks set to continue exerting its regulatory effects upon medicine, particularly in the areas of diagnosis and treatment, by discerning minimum standards of care from responsible customary practice, rather than from clinical guidelines.

Summary

Clinical guidelines can have an important role to play in situations where there is *both* considerable certainty about the best approach to treatment *and* where significant departure from such practice has no valid justification.

Uncritical adherence to clinical guidelines may lead to inappropriate clinical care.

Autonomous clinical thought is undermined by unthinking conformity to clinical guidelines.

Despite pressure from purchasers, rigid adherence to guidelines cannot be a formal managerial or legal expectation in the NHS.

References

1   Toulmin S (1993) Knowledge and art in the practice of medicine: clinical judgment and historical reconstruction. In: Delkeskamp-Hayes C and Gardell MA (eds) *Science, Technology and the Art of Medicine*. Cutter Kluwer Academic Publishers, Dordrecht, Boston and London, pp. 231–49.

2   Plato in: Annas J and Waterfield R (eds) (1995) *Statesman*. Cambridge University Press, Cambridge, pp. 59–77.

3   Carter A (1992) Clinical practice guidelines. *Can Med Assoc J*. **147**: 1649–50.

4   Plato in: Annas J and Waterfield R (eds) (1995) *Statesman*. Cambridge University Press, Cambridge, pp. xvi–xvii.

5   Plato in: translation by Saunders TJ (1970) *The Laws*. Penguin Books, London, pp. 181, 363.

6 Ellwood PM (1988) Outcomes management, a technology of patient experience. *NEJM*. **318**: 1549–56.

7 de Dombal FT (1987) Ethical considerations concerning computers in medicine in the 1980s. *J Medical Ethics*. **13**: 179–84.

8 Miller FG (1993) The concept of medically indicated treatment. *J Medicine and Philosophy*. **18**: 91–8.

9 Friedson E (1975) *Profession of Medicine*. Dodd Mead, New York.

10 Elstein AS, Lee SS and Sprafka SA (1978) *Medical Problem Solving*. Harvard University Press, Cambridge, MA, p. 23.

11 Feinstein AR (1994) Clinical judgment revisited: the distraction of quantitative models. *Ann Intern Med*. **120**: 799–805.

12 Gatens-Robinson E (1986) Clinical judgment and the rationality of the human sciences. *J Medicine and Philosophy*. **11**: 167–78.

13 Judson MA (1994) Clinical judgment. [Letter]. *Ann Intern Med*. **121**: 624.

14 Quoted by Wieland W (1993) The concept of the art of medicine. In: Delkeskamp-Hayes C and Gardell MA (eds) *Science, Technology and the Art of Medicine*. Cutter Kluwer Academic Publishers, Dordrecht, Boston and London, pp. 165–80.

15 McPherson K (1990) Why do variations occur? In: Anderson TF and Mooney G (eds) *The Challenge of Medical Practice Variations*. Macmillan, London, p. 17.

16 Havighurst C and King N (1983) Private credentialing of health care personnel: an antitrust perspective, Part I. *Am J Law Med*. **9**: 131–201.

17 Field M and Lohr K (1990) *Clinical Practice Guidelines: directions for a new program*. National Academy Press, Washington DC, p. 14.

18 Hirschfield EB (1991) Should practice parameters be the standard of care in malpractice litigation? *JAMA*. **226**: 2886–91.

19 McPherson K (1994) How should health policy be modified by the evidence of medical practice variations? In: Marinker M (ed.) *Controversies in Health Care Policies*. BMJ Publishing Group, London, pp. 55–74.

20 Williams A (1994) How should information on cost-effectiveness influence clinical practice? In: Delamothe T (ed.) *Outcomes into Clinical Practice*. BMJ Publishing Group, London, p. 100.

21 Hampton JR (1983) The end of clinical freedom. *BMJ*. **287**: 1237–8.

22 Hampton JR (1997) Evidence-based medicine, practice variations and clinical freedom. *J Evaluation in Clinical Practice*. **3**: 123–32.

23 Thompson SG and Pocock SJ (1991) Can meta-analysis be trusted? *Lancet.* **338**: 1127–30.

24 House of Lords Select Committee on Science and Technology (1995) *Minutes of Evidence taken before the Select Committee on Science and Technology.* Sub-committee 1. Medical Research and the NHS Reforms. HL Paper 12–iii: 151–67. HMSO, London.

25 Grimley Evans J (1995) Evidence-based and evidence-biased medicine. *Age and Ageing.* **24**: 461–3.

26 Greenhalgh T and Worrall J (1997) From EBM to CSM: the evolution of context sensitive medicine. *J Evaluation in Clinical Practice.* **3**: 105–8.

27 Hippocrates In: (1985) *The Genuine Works of Hippocrates.* The Classics of Medicine Library, AL, USA, p. 161.

28 Whitby L (1946) *The Science and Art of Medicine.* Cambridge University Press, Cambridge. Quoted in: Kessel N (1988) No more licence to practise. *Lancet.* i: 461 5.

29 Eddy DM (1993) Broadening the responsibilities of practitioners. *JAMA.* **269**: 1849–55.

30 McKee M and Clarke E (1995) Guidelines, enthusiasms, uncertainty and the limits to purchasing. *BMJ.* **310**: 101–4.

31 McCabe v Nassau County Medical Centre (United States Court of Appeals for the Second Circuit) (1971) **453** *Fed Reporter 2nd Series*: 698–709 at 708.

32 Grumet GW (1989) Health care rationing through inconvenience. *NEJM.* **321**: 607–11.

33 Downie RS and Charlton B (1992) *Medical Education in Theory and Practice.* Oxford University Press, Oxford, p. 181.

34 British Medical Association and the Law Society (1995) *Assessment of Mental Capacity: guidance for doctors and lawyers.* BMA, London.

35 Bolam v Friern Hospital Management Committee (1957) **2** *All ER*: 118–28 at 122.

36 Randall F and Downie RS (1996) *Ethics in Palliative Care.* Oxford University Press, Oxford, pp. 76–9.

37 Lomas J (1993) Making clinical policy explicit. *Int J Technol Assmt Hlth Care.* **9**: 11–25.

38 Dworkin R (1997) *Limits: the role of law in bioethical decision making.* Indiana University Press, Bloomington, IN, p. 3.

39 Nagel E (1985) Automation. In: Gardner M (ed.) *The Sacred Beetle.* Oxford University Press, Oxford, pp. 174–80.

40 See the case of F v R (1983) **33** *SASR*: 189.

41 Drife OJ (1989) Doctors, lawyers, and experts. *BMJ.* **299**: 746–7.

42 Medical Negligence Working Group (1995) *Lord Woolf's Inquiry: access to justice. Medical negligence litigation consultation paper.* Medical Negligence Working Group, London, pp. 24–8.
43 Lord Woolf (1997) Medics, lawyers and the courts. *J Roy Coll Phys London.* **31**: 686–93.
44 Eddy DM (1990) Clinical decision making from theory to practice. *JAMA.* **263**: 877–80.

Appendix 1
Key legal cases cited

Cases are listed chronologically by UK, Commonwealth and US jurisdiction.

United Kingdom cases

1953 *Crawford v Board of Governors of Charing Cross Hospital* (Court of Appeal) (*The Times*, 23 April and 8 December 1953; Mason J and McCall Smith R (eds) (1991) *Law and Medical Ethics*. Butterworths, London, p. 211)

This case turned upon whether there is a legally recognized onus upon doctors to be aware of recently published findings bearing upon the standard of care patients can expect from their doctor.

Mr Crawford, the plaintiff had been born with a useless left arm as a result of infantile paralysis. At the age of 52 he was admitted to hospital for a routine bladder operation which resulted in a severe right brachial palsy and a permanently useless right arm. The cause was prolonged abduction of the limb during the operation to allow free flow for an intravenous drip.

The judge in the lower court had found the anaesthetist involved to have been negligent. But this finding was later reversed by the Court of Appeal, which noted that the shoulder had been maintained at 80 degrees abduction throughout the procedure in accordance with customary practice at the time. In Lord Justice Somervell's view there was no evidence that the standard of care which Crawford received during the operation had departed from that which was customary at the time, and this excluded a finding of negligence.

In Somervell's view, the first judge had erred in basing his judgment on the aneasthetist's failure to read an article in the *Lancet* which had been published six months prior to the operation, pointing out the danger of brachial nerve palsy if an arm was kept in that degree of abduction for the period of time concerned in Crawford's operation. Lord Denning concurred:

'It would I think, be putting too high a burden on a medical man to say that he has to read every article appearing in the current medical press; and it would be quite wrong to suggest that the medical man is negligent because he does not at once put into operation the suggestion that some contributor or other might make in a medical journal. The time may come in a particular case when a new recommendation may be so well proved and so well known, and so well accepted that it should be adopted, but that was not so in this case.'

1955   *Hunter v Hanley*   (1955 Session Cases 200–8)

This is an influential Scottish medical negligence case in which the judge, Lord President Clyde, formulated the standard of medical care required by law in terms of the discretion doctors are to be allowed when deviating from customary care. Mrs Hunter was being treated for chronic bronchitis with a course of 12 injections of penicillin by Dr Hanley who used a size-16 needle. As Dr Hanley was withdrawing the twelfth injection, the needle broke and lodged in Mrs Hunter's body. The trial judge directed the jury that 'gross negligence' must be proved, but on appeal this was held to have been a mis-direction. Lord President Clyde said:

'In the realm of diagnosis and treatment there is ample scope for genuine difference of opinion and one man is not negligent merely because his conclusion differs from that of other professional men, nor because he has displayed less skill and knowledge than others would have shown. The true test in establishing negligence in diagnosis or treatment on the part of the doctor is whether he has been proved to be guilty of such failure as no doctor of ordinary skill would be guilty of if acting with ordinary care. The standard seems to be the same in England... To establish liability by a doctor where deviation from normal practice is alleged, three facts require to be established. First of all it must be proved that there is a normal practice; secondly it must be proved that the defendant has not adopted that practice; and thirdly (and this is of crucial importance) it must be established that the course the doctor adopted is one which no professional man of ordinary skill would have taken if he had been acting with ordinary care.'

1957   *Bolam v Friern Hospital Management Committee*   (1957 2 *All ER* 118–28)

This is the most influential formulation of the standard of medical care required by UK law which still holds sway over how cases of medical negligence, particularly with respect to diagnosis and treatment, are decided in UK courts.

John Hector Bolam sued Friern Hospital Management Committee claiming damages for negligence on their part, and on the part of their agents (i.e. staff), in administration of electro-convulsive treatment (ECT) which he had received in August 1954.

It was his second admission for a depressive illness that year, and he was advised to undergo ECT, for which he gave signed consent. He was not warned of the associated risks involved, including the risks of fracture. He underwent the first treatment on 19 August without incident. But as a result of the second treatment on 23 August, he sustained severe physical injuries including bilateral hip dislocations as a result of the femoral heads being driven medially through each pelvic acetabulum. John Bolam contended that the defendants were negligent in:

1 administering ECT without relaxant drugs or without manually constraining the resultant convulsive movements, and
2 in failing to warn him of the risk he was taking in consenting to the treatment.

The case came to court in February 1957. With respect to the first point, Judge McNair stated that competent doctors at the time apparently held divergent views about the desirability of using relaxant drugs, and about manually restraining the patient. One expert witness (for the plaintiff), a consultant psychiatrist, said he had used relaxant drugs selectively up to 1953, but after that time – a year before Mr Bolam's treatment – he had used relaxant drugs on *all* his patients and had never had a fracture. With respect to the importance of manual control the judge again found that there was a diversity of opinion. One expert witness believed it was foolhardy and substandard care in the absence of relaxant drugs not to provide manual restraint, but admitted that there was a competent body of medical opinion which maintained that the risk of fracture increased with the level of manual restraint. Other expert witnesses stated it was safer to hold the shoulders down and to allow the limbs to move – the practice which had been adopted at Friern from 1951 for administration of ECT with no obvious increase in fracture rate. The fracture rate from providing ECT without manual restraint quoted in court, and accepted by the judge, was 1 in 10 000. The judge reviewed the Accident and Emergency Department's fracture figures from Friern Hospital to confirm that there had been no increase in the fracture rates since manual restraint of the shoulders alone had been adopted at Friern. In Judge McNair's words:

'... where you get a situation which involves the use of some special skill or competence, then the test as to whether there has been negligence or not is not the test of the man on the top of the Clapham omnibus, because he has not got this special skill. The test is the standard of the ordinary skilled man exercising and professing to have that special skill. A man need not possess the highest expert skill; it is well established law that it is sufficient if he exercises the ordinary skill of an ordinary competent man exercising that particular art... A doctor is not guilty of negligence if he has acted in accordance with a practice accepted as proper by a responsible body of men skilled in that particular art... Putting it the other way round, a doctor is not negligent, if he is acting in accordance with such a practice, merely because there is a body of opinion that takes a contrary view...'

1985 *Gillick v West Norfolk and Wisbech Area Health Authority* (House of Lords) (1985 3 *All ER*: 402–37)

This action was started by Mrs Victoria Gillick following the publication, by the Department of Health and Social Security, of a memorandum of guidance as part of a 1981 circular (HSC(IS)32) concerning the provision of family planning in the National Health Service. The nub of Mrs Gillick's complaint was contained in a letter she wrote to the administrator of her local Area Health Authority:

'Concerning the *new* DHSS Guidelines on the contraceptive and abortion treatment of children under both the legal and medical age of consent... can I please ask you for a written assurance that in no circumstances whatsoever will any of my daughters... be given contraceptive or abortion treatment whilst they are under *sixteen*... without my knowledge, and irrefutable evidence of my consent?'

The reply she received from the chairman of the Area Health Authority displayed a clear appreciation of the relationship between guidance and clinical judgment:

'... it would be most unusual to provide advice about contraception without parental consent, but... the final decision must be for the doctor's clinical judgment. We would expect our doctors to work within these guidelines but, as the Minister has stated, the final decision in these matters must be one of clinical judgment.'

This was unacceptable to Mrs Gillick, and though the subsequent court action did not feature guidelines, it was notable for the view which the

House of Lords took on the capacity of a minor to consent to treatment despite parental objections. According to Lord Scarman:

'... the parental right to determine whether or not a minor child below the age of sixteen will have medical treatment terminates if and when the child achieves sufficient understanding and intelligence to enable him or her to understand fully what is being proposed.'

1986 *Wilsher v Essex Area Health Authority* (Court of Appeal) (1986 3 All ER: 801–38; Lexis transcript, Mead Data Central, OH)

This was a case in which the Court of Appeal had to consider whether a baby born three months prematurely, who suffered blindness from retrolental fibroplasia as a result of ventilation, did so because of negligent medical care.

The court at first instance had heard evidence about how arterial oxygen tensions were monitored in such babies, and about the levels considered safe and acceptable. The judge, Judge Pain, noted that the court had been 'favoured with an abundance of medical evidence as to these figures'. The case was referred to the Court of Appeal which reviewed both the pO_2 charts and the expert testimony produced at the original trial. The plaintiff's first witness, Dr Harvey, a consultant paediatrician at Queen Charlotte's Hospital, London, said he 'sensed danger the moment the needle read more than 12. Indeed, while he works at 8–12, he now prefers 7–11. He would not agree that the upper figure of 12 was merely a guideline'. The case shows how UK courts set about considering claims and weighing expert testimony in actions alleging medical negligence, in which the notion of a guideline can be invoked as an entirely permissive piece of advice or a minimum standard of care.

1987 *Dally v The General Medical Council (Privy Council)* (Lexis transcript, Mead Data Central, OH)

Allegedly failing to follow 'guidelines laid down for good clinical practice' when prescribing methadone and other drugs was one of six separate allegations made by the GMC against Dr Ann Dally. The GMC contended that she had issued prescriptions for the drugs irresponsibly and was therefore guilty of serious professional misconduct.

Dr Dally appealed to the Privy Council against the findings of the GMC's Professional Conduct Committee which had not found her guilty of any of the six allegations of the first charge, but had determined that she was guilty of serious professional misconduct on a second charge, that of issuing such prescriptions to a Mr 'A' without conducting a proper examination of the patient, and without adequately monitoring his progress, a charge which the Privy Council upheld.

1988 *McFarlane v Secretary of State for Scotland* (1988 Scottish Civil LR: 623–8)

Courts may not accept mechanistic applications of a guideline or recommendation, as this appeal to a sheriff against revocation of a driving licence shows. Rather, courts expect expert practitioners – in this case administrators   at   the   appropriate   licensing   authority   –   to *interpret* a guideline's significance in the context of individual circumstances.

Despite the recommendations of the Council of Ophthalmologists and of their advisory panel to the Secretary of State for Transport, that the minimum visual field for safe driving should include a 20 degree width above and below the horizontal, and the uncontested finding in the case of the appellant, Mr McFarlane, that his field of vision did not amount to such a width, the sheriff nevertheless found him fit to drive on the evidence of expert witnesses.

The sheriff noted that although the Secretary of State's advisers had given the case 'most careful consideration', they had 'simply followed the recommendations in the guidelines laid down'. Further expert testimony focused upon the congenital nature of the appellant's visual defect, which was neither degenerative nor progressive, and to which he had fully adapted. He suffered from a left upper homonymous quadrantanopia which the sheriff deemed would be of little significance to a driver looking straight ahead, or from side to side in the rear mirror. He was not thought to be a danger to the public and his licence was duly reinstated.

1989 *In: Re F (Mental patient: sterilization)* (1989 2 WLR: 1025–62)

A key case heard by the House of Lords in which the Law Lords outlined two roles for guidelines:

1 to assist doctors in taking difficult ethical decisions when treating incompetent adults and
2 to provide doctors with a degree of legal protection.

The case concerned a 36-year old severely mentally handicapped woman with the mental age of a small child, who, while living in a mental hospital as a voluntary patient, had formed a sexual relationship with a male patient. Her mother and the hospital staff believed F lacked any concept of pregnancy or birth, and considered that she would be unable to cope with the effects of pregnancy and giving birth, the psychiatric consequences of which it was alleged would be 'catastrophic' for F.

All forms of contraception were considered highly undesirable, and it was thought to be wrong to restrict her freedom, and prevent her sexual activity. Her mother sought and was granted a declaration from the court that F's sterilization would be in her best interests, and would not be unlawful by reason of the absence of the patient's consent, despite the fact that sterilization did not amount to a therapeutic procedure. The Court of Appeal upheld the lower court's decision as did the House of Lords.

Much of the case report is taken up with complex legal arguments concerning where the jurisdiction is to be found in UK law to consent to bodily invasion in the case of incompetent adults. The judges acknowledged the difficulty of deciding the correct course of action, and acknowledged the associations which arose from the case with eugenics and the Nazi sterilization programmes.

The judges were in no doubt about the legal risks which doctors face in administering various treatments to incompetent patients. In the leading judgment, Lord Donaldson stated that:

'consultation with other doctors and with those in other caring disciplines may be necessary if the doctor... is to be able to satisfy himself, and it may be subsequently a court, that he is performing his duty under the law and so is immune from suit. This difficulty of decision cannot ever be removed, but it would undoubtedly be much lessened if the medical profession were to produce ethical and professional guidelines for the treatment of incompetent adults,'

a point reiterated by Lords Justice Butler Sloss and Neill.

1989 W v Edgell   (1989 1 All ER: 1089–109; 1990 9 WLR: 474–93)

W had killed four people and had been convicted of manslaughter ten years previously on the grounds of diminished responsibility. He was detained in a secure hospital.

W sought an injunction against the Home Secretary and others to prevent them disclosing or using a report prepared at the request of W's solicitors by a pyschiatrist, Dr Edgell. The report was unfavourable towards W in his application to a mental health tribunal considering his discharge or transfer to a regional secure unit. On receipt of Dr Edgell's report, W's solicitors had withdrawn the application to the tribunal.

Although Dr Edgell had been asked to examine W solely to provide the patient and his solicitors with his assessment, he saw fit to send a copy of his report to W's hospital which forwarded it on to the Home Secretary and to the tribunal. W claimed that Edgell had breached his duty of confidentiality towards him. However, the judge at first instance found that the circumstances of the case fell squarely within the GMC's guidelines (referred to as 'rules' in the judgment), as laid out in its *Advice on Standards of Professional Conduct and Medical Ethics*, which permit doctors to disclose confidential medical information to other doctors with clinical responsibility for a patient's care. This view was affirmed by the Court of Appeal although Lord Justice Bingham expressed some reservations.

1990   *Loveday v Renton and Wellcome Foundation Ltd*   (1990 1 Med LR: 117–86)

This case provides a good illustration of how UK civil courts decide issues of medical fact and medical negligence. The case concerned a baby girl who suffered brain damage after receiving a pertussis vaccination, despite coming within the then current contraindications issued by the Department of Health. In addition to the main question which the court had to decide, namely, whether pertussis vaccine could cause brain damage, it was submitted by the plaintiff that:

'a doctor who vaccinated in breach of contraindications (guidelines issued to doctors on vaccination procedures) was negligent and would be liable for any resulting brain damage [original parentheses].'

In the context of expert testimony provided to the court, the judge carefully reviewed all the statements of advice issued by the Department of Health from 1963 onwards, together with that provided by the American Academy of Paediatrics in 1986.

It was held that failure to observe the contraindication guidelines did 'not in itself constitute negligence because there was a respectable and responsible body of medical opinion that some contraindications should not be observed because the risk of disease outweighed any actual or possible risk from the vaccine'.

Although this finding was *obiter*, i.e. not central to the main issue which the court had to decide, namely whether whooping cough vaccine *could* cause brain damage, the judge issued the ruling specifically in order to 'give guidance to future litigants on the assumption that the plaintiff succeeds on the issue of causation' (which in fact she did not).

The judgment is interesting for its explication of the relationship between written guidelines, expert testimony presented to the court, and the opinions of unnamed respectable others:

'In so far as the plaintiff seeks to rely on the contraindications as evidence of the opinions of experts not called as witnesses that the vaccine can cause brain damage, this evidence is inadmissible in law. The reason for this is obvious; it is not known who holds the opinion or basis of it; and the evidence is not tested in cross-examination before the court. It is hearsay. But it is part of the medical literature in the case, experts are entitled to and have commented on it...

The question of whether the vaccine can cause brain damage is not answered by showing that there is a respectable and responsible body of medical opinion that the vaccine can, albeit rarely, cause permanent brain damage, or that this view may be more widely held than the contrary... The works of learned and qualified authors form part of the general corpus of medical and scientific learning on the subject and can be relied upon and adopted by suitably qualified experts. These experts may have their opinions tested in the light of this literature.'

1992   In: Re W (a minor)   (1992 3 WLR: 758–82)

This case, heard before the Court of Appeal, involved a 16-year old competent minor with anorexia nervosa who refused treatment in a specialist centre. The court at first instance authorized treatment without W's consent, notwithstanding the then current Department of Health's *Guidelines for Ethics Committees* (1991) which stated: 'The giving of consent by a parent or guardian cannot override a refusal of consent by a child who is competent to make that decision'. The elaborate arguments of Lord Donaldson in the Court of Appeal, which upheld the original decision, are sometimes difficult to follow, but clearly demonstrate that courts are free to disagree with guidelines drawn up by authoritative bodies such as the Department of Health, especially where a point of law is concerned.

1993   *Airedale NHS Trust v Bland* (House of Lords)   (1993 1 *All ER*: 821–96)

This case involved a decision by doctors caring for Tony Bland, a patient in a persistent vegetative state (PVS), to withdraw hydration and nutrition from him thereby allowing him to die.

The case arose because the NHS Trust responsible for his care applied to the High Court for a declaration to the effect that the proposed course of action would be proper and lawful. The declaration granted by the court at first instance was affirmed by the Court of Appeal and by the House of Lords. The courts decided that withdrawal of nutrition in a case of PVS amounted to discontinuation of medical treatment, which could only be lawful if it was judged to be in the patient's best interests. Although their Lordships disagreed about whether a patient in PVS could meaningfully be said to have any interests at all, they decided that further treatment could serve no useful purpose, and in the view of one judge could amount legally to battery (unconsented touching).

The leading judgment in the House of Lords was given by Lord Goff who elaborated the safeguards which must be observed before discontinuation of life support in cases of PVS. He approved of the guidelines which had been developed by the Medical Ethics Committee of the British Medical Association designed to ensure both reliability of diagnosis and ethically appropriate treatment of patients with PVS:

'Study of this document left me in no doubt that, if a doctor treating a PVS patient acts in accordance with the medical practice now being evolved by the Medical Ethics Committee of the BMA, he will be acting with the benefit of guidance from a responsible and competent body of professional opinion, as required by the *Bolam* test.'

1994   *Ratty v Haringey Health Authority and another* (Court of Appeal)   (1995 5 *Med LR*: 413–21; Lexis manuscript, Mead Data Central, OH)

A case illustrating that even an apparently simple guideline may yet be equivocal in meaning and ambiguous in application. The plaintiff underwent an abdomino-perineal resection (APR) for a stenosing lesion of the sigmoid colon, though there was no biopsy proof of cancer. At operation, 'a huge mass was found in the pelvis infiltrating the bladder and involving the bladder' and the surgeon proceeded to full APR. Subsequent histology proved that the mass was not cancer. The plaintiff claimed it was irresponsible in any circumstances to perform an APR without prior proof of a malignant lesion, and sought to back this position up with reference to 'Marnham's Rule'. This rule, attributed to the surgeon Sir Ralph Marnham, asserts that an APR should only be performed when there is histological proof of cancer.

The court at first instance agreed with him, found negligence on the part of the surgeons concerned, and awarded substantial damages against the health authority. The Court of Appeal noted that one expert witness had himself performed an APR 'more than once when he had what he regarded as sufficient clinical evidence of cancer without having available histological proof'. 'Marnham's Rule', according to two of the expert witnesses, was only 'a useful guideline, but not one to be followed in every case'. Since these surgeons represented a responsible and reputable body of opinion in colo-rectal surgery, Lord Justice Kennedy ruled that the court at first instance should not have accepted the plaintiff's formulation of 'Marnham's Rule' when evaluating the conduct of the defendant surgeon, but should have accepted the view of two responsible expert surgeon's concerning its status as 'a useful guideline' only, which required reasonable interpretation.

1994 *Early v Newham Health Authority* (1994 *5 Med LR*: 214–17)

The plaintiff, a 13-year old girl, alleged that an intubation protocol approved by a health authority was faulty. She had awoken whilst still paralysed from suxamethonium, and argued that the protocol followed in her treatment, which advised insufflation of the lungs with oxygen rather than an oxygen-anaesthetic mixture was faulty; she claimed it would be likely to allow a patient to regain consciousness whilst still paralysed, thereby causing unnecessary injury through fright and distress.

The judge was advised on the origin of the protocol and its use in hospitals in the UK and abroad. Notwithstanding the testimony of a professor of anaesthesia that '... no reasonably competent medical authority would have condoned this drill', the judge found in favour of the defendants. He judged the authors of the protocol to be a competent body of medical practitioners who had adopted a prevalent protocol in a responsible manner. He held that:

'Unless a medical procedure is patently unsafe or goes against common practice or usage a court should not attempt to substitute its views for those of the profession.'

1995   *Vernon v Bloomsbury Health Authority*   (1995 **6** *Med LR*: 297–310)

The plaintiff, Barbara Vernon, was treated in University College Hospital in 1982 for culture negative bacterial endocarditis. She received doses of gentamycin higher than those recommended by the *Product Data Sheet*, the *British National Formulary* (*BNF*), the *Monthly Index of Medical Specialities* (*MIMS*) and *Martindale's Extra Pharmacopoiea*, and for a period longer than that recommended by *MIMS* and *Martindale's*. She had been given 5.625 mg/kg for 19 days, whereas these reference sources recommended a maximum dose of 5 mg/kg for seven days. She recovered from the endocarditis but suffered bilateral vestibular damage and loss of balance as a result.

Judge Tucker heard from several expert witnesses, all but one of whom said that they themselves would have prescibed gentamycin at this dosage for a patient in Barbara Vernon's condition. One of the plaintiff's expert witnesses stated that she would not have administered such a high dose for a patient in such a condition, but she was unable to say that no reasonably competent microbiologist could prescribe at this level. The judge found that:

'... the dosage was a proper one. The doctors were not negligent in prescribing it. I agree with the defendants' experts that the guidelines laid down by the manufacturers and, for example, MIMS, are too conservative and that they err on the side of caution. I accept the views expressed by Dr Sowton, Dr Reeves and Dr Cooke, all of whom have great practical experience of prescribing this drug. In particular, I rely on the views of Dr Reeves. He has consistently prescribed higher doses than those recommended by the manufacturers and has advised others to do the same.'

Commonwealth cases

1991   *Re X*   (1991 **2** *New Zealand LR*: 365–78)

In this case, the judge quoted the views of the Medical Council of New Zealand, concerning the role of guidelines in helping to ensure that doctors properly inform patients about the nature of their medical condition and any proposed treatment:

'In judging whether the medical practitioner has fallen short of acceptable practice in these matters, disciplinary authorities should have recourse to guidelines that are published from time to time... The Council does not believe that these guidelines should themselves be enacted in legislative form, however it supports the view that legislation should ensure that any definition of medical misconduct should include the inadequate transfer of information to a patient deciding on a medical procedure.'

1992 *Cranley v Medical Board of Western Australia* (1992 3 *Med LR*: 94–113)

This case was an appeal to the Supreme Court of Western Australia by an Australian general practitioner against the Australian Medical Board which in 1990 had found him guilty of 'infamous' and 'improper conduct' in pursuing a 'harm reduction policy' in his treatment of drug addicts. Dr Cranley had been charged with contravening the *Australian National Methadone Guidelines*, and with prescribing injectable diazepam ampoules for self-administration for which it was alleged there could never be any clinical indications. The Board had held that 'the prescribing of drugs for purposes other than pharmacologically to reduce dependence on heroin, or alleviate withdrawal symptoms, was, in effect, improper because such purposes were not "therapeutic"'. The Board decided that Dr Cranley had not 'adhered to the orthodox method of treatment' which at the time restricted prescriptions to oral preparations, available only at specialist units. The Supreme Court reversed the finding because it found that there was indeed a minority medical view, reputable and respectable, which approved of a harm reduction policy and that, moreover, the *Australian National Metha-done Guidelines* could be understood as reflecting a broad harm reduction policy that did not interdict the prescribing of parenteral diazepam. If a court or tribunal fails to acknowledge the legitimacy of a possible plurality of approaches to the medical care of a condition it is likely to be over-ruled by a higher court.

United States cases

1971 *McCabe v Nassau County Medical Center* (1971 **453** *Fed Reporter 2d Series*: 698–709)

In this case, heard by a US Court of Appeals, a 25-year old married woman with four children had been refused a sterilization procedure at her local public hospital because the regulations of Nassau County Medical Center used an age-parity formula at that time, derived from the recommendations of the American College of Obstetricians and Gynaecologists. These stated that a woman of this age needed to have five living children to be eligible for voluntary sterilization. Mrs McCabe brought an action alleging that the hospital's refusal to sterilize her infringed her constitutional rights. The case is noteworthy for the view expressed by the judge concerning the undesirability of such guidelines:

'Fortunately for our society, the State has wisely not undertaken to establish medical guidelines and procedures for doctors and surgeons in public hospitals. Of all professions in which the exercise of judgment should be as uncontrolled as possible, it is the medical profession.'

1974   *Helling v Carey*   (1974 **519** *Pacific Reporter 2d Series*: 981–5)

In this much debated US case, two ophthalmologists were successfully sued for failure to diagnose glaucoma before loss of vision in a woman aged 32. They had frequently examined the plaintiff over the previous nine years for refraction and contact lens assessments. The court at first instance entered judgment for the defendant doctors after receiving uncontroverted testimony that 'the standards of the profession for that speciality do not require pressure tests for glaucoma upon patients under 40'. It is noteworthy that this court relied entirely upon expert testimony to establish customary practice. No references to professionally developed guidelines, or recommendations from a recognized association of ophthalmologists were put before the court. The Supreme Court of the State of Washington reversed the lower court's decision, holding that:

'Irrespective of... the standards of the ophthalmology profession... as a matter of law... the reasonable standard that should have been followed... was the timely giving of this simple, harmless pressure test.'

The Supreme Court quoted a famous pronouncement of Justice Hand: 'Courts must in the end say what is required; there are precautions so imperative that even their universal disregard will not excuse their omission.' The decision, which has not been generally followed, illustrates the power of courts in common law jurisdictions to set minimum standards of medical care, albeit in this instance, in the context of the provision of a screening test. The rationale of the decision appears to be that people under 40 are entitled to the same protection, in the court's view, as the older age group. The ruling was controversial at the time because in order to detect *one* case of glaucoma by tonometric screening of the under 40 age group, 25 000 people would need to be tested, and follow-up arranged for potentially large numbers of false negatives, false positives and borderline cases. Despite the astronomical costs involved in substituting this judicial standard of care for one based upon customary medical practice, the Supreme Court did not hesitate to reiterate its position in a later case alleging negligent treatment of iritis. In *Harris v Robert C Groth* (1983) it was stated that:

'The standard of care against which a health care provider's conduct is to be measured is that of a reasonably prudent practitioner possessing the degree of skill, care, and learning possessed by other members of the profession in the state of Washington. The degree of care actually practiced by members of the profession is only some evidence of what is reasonably prudent – it is not dispositive.'

1977 *Rodriguez v Jackson* (1977 574 *Pacific Reporter* 2d *Series*: 481–6)

This case was heard in the Arizona Court of Appeal. Rodriguez contended that the vestibular damage he suffered as a result of streptomycin therapy for pulmonary tuberculosis occurred as a result of negligence on the part of his physician who had administered four times the dose recommended by a manual entitled *The Tuberculosis Control Program in Arizona, March 1969*. The judges noted that the manual was designed to provide the practitioner with guidelines for the diagnosis, treatment and prevention of clinical tuberculosis, but ruled that it did not set a standard of care the breach of which constituted malpractice. While the manual was admissible as evidence, such guidelines do not represent conclusive evidence of the customary standard of care.

1986 *Lowry v Henry Mayo Newhall Memorial Hospital* (1986 229 *Cal Rptr*: 620–5)

This report concerns a malpractice suit brought against a physician on behalf of a woman alleging that she had been 'arbitrarily' given atropine but not adrenaline which was the drug recommended by the American Heart Association's guidelines for advanced cardiac life support and resuscitation procedure. The woman had been admitted to hospital following a road traffic accident and then suffered a cardiac arrest. Summary judgment was made for the defendant doctor after she successfully maintained that the American Heart Association guidelines were 'mere guidelines that may be altered by the physician'. The judgment was termed 'summary' because the plaintiff had failed to raise a triable issue of fact, the case being viewed as 'entirely without merit on any legal theory'. The California Court of Appeal confirmed the judgment.

1986 *Wickline v State of California* (1986 **228** Cal Rptr: 661–72)

This case involved early discharge of a patient according to a Medi-Cal protocol consisting of treatment guidelines, including length of stay criteria approved for payment purposes. It was alleged that as a result of too early a discharge, the patient had to undergo an amputation and that the physician who had allowed the discharge to take place had thereby been negligent. The doctor had not protested against the protocol because he believed a request for extended hospitalization would have been refused by the payer. Expert testimony in court stated that the doctor's decision to allow discharge, at the time when he did, fell within the boundaries of the customary standard of care. He was therefore not found liable in negligence. However, the court held that there was an obligation upon a physician, in circumstances in which a patient's condition could benefit from further hospitalization, to appeal for an extension of hospital stay, even if such extension was likely to have been refused. The court did not go on to consider whether Medi-Cal's review criteria were defective or whether it had breached a duty of care to the patient. The court emphasized, however, that:

'a patient who is harmed when care which should have been provided and is not provided should recover [*damages*]... from all those responsible for the deprivation of care, including, when appropriate, health care payors.'

The ruling implies that if a patient comes to harm as a result of the implementation of review criteria and guidelines for length of hospital stay, the guideline promulgators may in principle be held liable. In addition, a physician cannot defend himself against a charge of negligence by claiming that his own judgment was swayed and corrupted by defective guidelines or protocols.

1988 *James v Wooley* (1988 **523** *Southern Reporter 2d Series*: 110–13)

This case was an appeal against summary judgment by a lower court, which had found in favour of defendant doctors in a medical malpractice action in which the plaintiff, a baby, had been born with a paretic arm. Its mother was obese (5 feet 4 inches tall and 316 pounds in weight), and suffered from gestational diabetes and hypertension, and the baby had presented with shoulder dystocia. It was alleged that the mother's doctors had been negligent in opting for vaginal delivery and that the baby should have been delivered instead by caesarian section. The Supreme Court of Alabama reversed the original ruling in favour of the doctors and sent the dispute for a jury trial after hearing the testimony of an expert witness:

'Anytime a woman, particularly a gestational diabetic, is estimated to have a baby in excess of 4000 grams, a cesarian section should be done. Here, by the way, I am quoting from the technical bulletin of the *American College of Obstetricians and Gynecologists*.'

The court found this testimony and its reference to accepted guidelines raised the possibility that an accepted standard of care had been breached:

'These statements create a genuine issue of material fact requiring resolution by a jury. While it strains credibility to suggest that the weight of the baby is the single determining factor when a physician must decide between a vaginal and a cesarian delivery, it is not a function of the Court to pass on the credibility of the witnesses. This function is reserved for the jury.'

1990 *Wilson v Blue Cross of Southern California* (1990 **271** *Cal Rptr 3rd Series*: 876–85)

The Appeal Court of California held that a doctor's failure to protest against inappropriate review rules in the case of a patient harmed by adherence to these rules did not automatically protect the review organization from liability in negligence. The case involved a depressed patient who committed suicide after early discharge from hospital as a result of a decision by Blue Cross, through its agents, Western Medical, to refuse payment for further hospital care. The court found that 'Western Medical's decision not to approve further hospitalization was a substantial factor in bringing about the decedent's demise'. The court also stated its view that: 'The language in *Wickline v State of California* which suggests that civil liability for a discharge decision rests solely within the responsibility of a treating physician is *dicta*' that is, not a necessary part of the decision itself; it does not therefore set a precedent binding upon other courts.

1996 *Snyder v American Association of Blood Banks* (1996 676 *Atlantic Reporter 2d Series*: 1036–64)

In this case, it was alleged that the American Association of Blood Banks (AABB), a trade association of voluntary blood banks, was liable to a patient for omitting to advise its member blood bank associations to institute measures to lessen the likelihood of AIDS transmission by blood transfusion. In 1984, William Snyder had received an HIV infected blood transfusion supplied by Bergen Community Blood Center and subsequently he developed AIDS. He contended that the AABB had been negligent in failing to recommend the screening of donors by way of surrogate testing prior to August 1984. The initial court had found for the plaintiff, but the AABB appealed on the grounds that it was a third party with no immediate responsibility for patient care, and did not have a duty of care towards Mr Snyder.

The court noted that in 1983 the Centers for Disease Control Task Force had concluded that AIDS was very likely to be transmissible in blood. The Task Force had therefore recommended techniques for screening out high-risk blood donors, by detailed questioning about past history and life-style and by surrogate testing of collected blood. Though not made compulsory by the Federal Drugs Agency at the time, some blood banks had adopted these procedures but in 1983 the AABB had rejected the advice on the grounds of cost.

The court recognized that the AABB had no direct involvement in obtaining or processing the blood used to transfuse Mr Snyder, but held that by 1983 it should have foreseen that transfusions could transmit AIDS. The AABB had a leading position in setting minimum standards in a self-governing industry; its role in controlling and accrediting member institutions meant that its members were reliant upon it for instituting safe and appropriate standards for blood quality, and this gave rise to a duty of care to patients. The court therefore affirmed the AABB's negligence.

Appendix 2
Selected further reading: legal
significance of clinical guidelines

References and annotations are listed by author, under the jurisdiction to which they mainly refer.

United Kingdom

• Chalmers I (1994) Why are opinions about the effects of health care so often wrong? *Medico-Legal Journal*. **62**: 116–30.

Transcript of a talk given by the Director of the UK Cochrane Centre to the Medico-Legal Society in November 1993. The author discusses concerns about the wide gap which exists in many areas of clinical practice between established medical policies (opinion-based guidelines) and evidence-based practice. Unfortunately no references are provided. Good points are made in the discussion which follows by Brahams, Morrison and Leigh

• Harpwood V (1994) NHS reform, audit, protocols and standards of care. *Medical Law International*. **1**: 241–59.

This paper critically examines the limitations of the Bolam principle in the context of the law of negligence, the post-1990 NHS reforms and recent moves towards protocol-informed health care.

• Holyoak J (1990) Raising the standard of care. *Legal Studies*. **10**: 210–11.

A careful consideration of common law negligence actions showing that compliance with customary clinical practice is not always a sure defence to a charge of negligence, particularly where the courts in common law jurisdictions find 'obvious folly'. As the author makes clear, negligence by all is no defence to negligence. Notwithstanding the Bolam test, it is the courts which have the last say over what constitutes negligence. Holyoak shows that the courts, by substituting their own standard for that customarily adopted in practice, may seek to *raise* the standard of care required from professionals.

● Hurwitz B (1994) Clinical guidelines: proliferation and medicolegal significance. *Quality in Health Care*. **3**: 37–44.
● Hurwitz B (1995) Protocols, guidelines and the law of negligence. *Clinical Risk*. **1**: 142–6.
● Hurwitz B (1995) Clinical guidelines and the law: advice, guidance or regulation? *J Evaluation in Clinical Practice*. **1**: 49–60.

A series of articles addressing the possible roles of clinical guidelines as instruments of health care regulation.

● Kennedy I (1993) Medicine in society, now and in the future. In: Lock S (ed.) *Eighty-Five Not Out: essays to honour Sir George Godber*. King Edward's Hospital Fund For London, London, pp. 69–75.

A discussion by a distinguished professor of medical law of how the shift towards providing, purchasing and consuming health care within the NHS inevitably brings with it greater recourse to the law as a means of enforcing accountability. Professor Kennedy sees protocols and guidelines as explicit manifestations of accountability at work, and he believes they will inevitably make a contribution to defining whether treament decisions are fair and lawful.

● Stern K (1995) Clinical guidelines and negligence liability. In: Deighan M and Hitch S (eds) *Clinical Effectiveness: from guidelines to cost-effective practice*. Earlybrave Publications Ltd, Brentwood, pp. 127–35.

The author clearly outlines the regulatory roles of clinical guidelines and their possible relevance in actions alleging negligence.

Commonwealth

• Jutras D (1993) Clinical practice guidelines as practice norms. *Can Med Assoc J*. **148**: 905–8.

The author, Professor of Law from McGill University, explores whether clinical guidelines which are generally developed with a view to improving the quality of health care, could nevertheless be viewed as legal norms expressing 'relevant legal standard(s) of care'. If this were so, the author believes that screening complaints using guideline norms could cut down the number of frivolous claims and, conversely, promote more court actions in cases likely to succeed. Guidelines could also help judges and juries to be more consistent in their decisions as to what kind of care constitutes negligence. Other than by passing a statute or regulation stating that a given guideline constitutes a legal standard of care, and in the absence of contractual agreements between doctors and patients to the effect that treatment will only be given in compliance with certain guidelines, clinical guidelines can only approach the status of a legal norm if the courts so decide. The authority and disinterest of guideline developers, the methodologies adopted, the extensiveness of guideline adoption, and their actual use within the relevant medical community, are all factors likely to weigh heavily with a court in deciding whether guidelines can be treated as legal norms. To the extent that guidelines are often put forward with a view to *changing* practice, rather than codifying existing practices, they are unlikely to play a *decisive* role in litigation. This is probably the best introductory article to the legal issues surrounding guidelines, though it provides few examples of legal cases.

• Lomas J (1993) Making clinical policy explicit. *Int J Technol Ass Hlth Care*. **9**: 11–25.

The author uses the analogy between formation of clinical policy and legislative policy-making to highlight the relative immaturity of clinical guideline development techniques. Practice guidelines in Lomas's view should be viewed as 'policies insofar as a policy is a rule to establish, control, or change the behaviour of institutions, individuals, or both'. The creation of clinical guidelines, the author argues, requires to be seen and analysed as a policy-making activity within society. Until recently, much clinical policy-making has been accomplished informally, by unwritten processes not open to public (or even wide professional) debate, and frequently without a clear strategy for implementation or 'enforcement'. Lomas believes that the relatively primitive and under-developed policy-making processes of clinical medicine have much to gain from a study of public policy legislation, which by contrast is usually 'written, debated in public, developed through a formal process, and has official instruments of enforcement or implementation'. The legislative process, having evolved in order to express, to some degree, a democratic wish to limit and overcome the unfettered power of a sovereign or colonial ruler to *impose* policy upon a people, necessarily involves:

'accountability and responsivity to available estimates of the facts (evidence), interested parties' interpretations of facts (vested interests), and the relative priorities afforded to the facts (values).'

The author outlines the steps involved in explicit policy-making, and uses his own work on creating and implementing clinical policy for caesarian section to illustrate the process. He contends that valid and accepted practice guidelines have become for medicine:

'what legislative statutes have for years been for governments – the embodiment of the best available solutions to the prevalent problems in an explicit format that is accountable to all the parties of interest.'

The paper offers an evocative and thoughtful analysis of the many policy issues raised by clinical guideline proliferation.

United States

• Ayres JD (1994) The use and abuse of medical practice guidelines. *J Legal Medicine*. 15: 421–43.

This paper provides a broad review of the place of medical practice guidelines in modern clinical practice. Written by a legally qualified assistant professor of medicine, it focuses upon the strengths and weaknesses of different development strategies, the evolving relationship between research evidence and clinical guidelines, and sources of bias to which guideline creation processes are subject. The author emphasizes the dangers of confusing guidelines with model standards of care:

'the potential for such bias should be sufficient to slow down the drive to apply practice parameters in malpractice litigation by 'judicial notice' or to apply them as 'standards of care' in any proposed alternative dispute resolution system or litigation.'

Reference to court decisions are few in this paper, which seems to have been written to inform lawyers of the medical background to practice guidelines rather than to inform doctors as to how the legal process might seek to make use of guidelines.

● Brennan TA (1991) Practice guidelines and malpractice litigation: collision or cohesion? *J Health Politics Policy and Law*. **16**: 67–85.

This paper provides a wide ranging review of the evolving role of practice guidelines in US malpractice suits. Rules of evidence together with the US hearsay and locality rules which govern introduction of guidelines into court are clearly stated. In the author's view, guidelines will increasingly feature in malpractice litigation, though they are unlikely to fundamentally transform the manner in which the courts determine negligence.

● Garnick DW, Hendricks AM and Brennan TA (1991) Can practice guidelines reduce the number and costs of malpractice claims? *JAMA*. **266**: 2856–60.

This paper presents many of the legal issues surrounding practice guidelines in the USA in a form accessible to a medical readership. The authors argue that practice guidelines are unlikely to reduce the number or the costs of malpractice in the USA for the following reasons: probably less than 20% of malpractice cases relate to specific conditions or occurrences to which guidelines apply; many guidelines are not widely accepted and do not represent customary practice which is still the mainstay standard of care adopted in US malpractice suits; until effective guidelines are integrated into routine clinical practice their potential to improve the quality of medical care through consequent reduction in patient harm is unlikely to be translated into fewer law suits. Guidelines are usually designed to be flexible, allowing varying degrees of discretion on the part of users, so a degree of deviation from such guidelines cannot simply imply malpractice. Guidelines will not dispense with the role of expert witnesses who will continue to be required to help courts to:

'(1) establish that members of the profession consider a particular practice guideline to be authoritative; (2) propose an alternate standard of care that might apply (e.g. articles, recent research, local institutional guidelines, or a different practice guideline); (3) provide reasons why a defendant should not have followed the guideline in a particular case; (4) argue that the practice guideline is not applicable to a plaintiff's case; (5) debate the weight to be given to competing guidelines from different sources; and (6) affirm that guidelines are up-to-date and reflect changes in practice and increased scientific knowledge.'

• Havighurst CC (1990) Practice guidelines for medical care: the policy rationale. *St Louis Univ Law J.* **34**: 777–819.

The author, a professor of law, views guidelines as regulatory instruments for improving standards which doctors, patients, payers and courts look to for authoritative guidance on the appropriateness of medical treatments. In the author's view, control of guideline creation and content is a political issue. The medical profession's attempt to develop and capture guideline development reflects its agenda of retaining the power to set norms and standards for itself, thereby maintaining clinical autonomy within self-defined parameters. A challenge to this model has come from pressure to include non-medical interests in guideline development such as patient preference and cost considerations. These developments hold out the possibility that treatment guidelines will come to express a wider set of values than those held by doctors alone. However, the author believes that by synthesizing the results of *conflicting* health care studies and teachings into one authoritative guideline, clinical guidelines are generally exerting too much regulation upon health care. He argues that the main role for practice guidelines should be to meet the information requirements of a de-regulated health care system, allowing patients, payers and others to choose their health care from a variety of guidelines expressing *different*, though considered, judgments about scientific evidence, marginal benefits and debatable health issues. A multiplicity of treatment guidelines developed outside the auspices of the medical profession would allow patients and contractors a much greater say in the type and standard of treatments on offer from doctors. The author calls for pluralism to be built into the US Federal guidelines programme.

• Havighurst CC (1991) Practice guidelines as legal standards governing physician liability. *Law and Contemporary Problems.* **54**: 87–117.

The author provides a clear exposition of the possible ways that US practice guidelines can influence the standard of medical care required in actions alleging medical negligence: by a guideline providing evidence as to customary care; because it purports to set a standard of care (in which case further evidence that a guideline was *in fact* influential would be sought by a court); because a particular guideline has been developed by a prestigious organization which itself is influential in setting the standard of care; because legislation can direct courts to treat guidelines 'not merely as evidence of the standard of care but as the standard itself'.

● Hirschfield EB (1991) Should practice parameters be the standard of care in malpractice litigation? *JAMA.* **226**: 2886–91.

The author considers whether US common law should be altered to require courts to apply practice guidelines or parameters as the standard of care in cases of alleged medical negligence. He notes that state legislation in Maine already provides such a framework, and alludes to federal bills in varying degrees of preparation which, if passed, could make similar provision in different legal settings. He argues that there is, as yet, insufficient common understanding of the different characteristics of clinical guidelines, and because of the danger of promoting guideline development in areas of medical practice in which diversity of approach remains desirable, such a move would be premature. He notes that successful and effective guidelines may display very different characteristics, as he illustrates in comparing a practice parameter developed by the American Society of Anesthesiologists designed to ensure adequate partial pressure of oxygen is maintained during operations, with that developed by the American College of Cardiologists which aimed to cut down inappropriate pacemaker insertions. The first parameter applies to almost all operations without exception, whereas the second divides patients into several categories depending upon underlying diagnosis, the absence, presence and severity of certain symptoms, and includes at least one grey area category of uncertainty. He argues that the first parameter, which covers an area of certainty, is inherently more suited to become a legal standard than the second parameter which is much more complex, and seeks to manage varying degrees of certainty. Areas of uncertainty are also generally areas of research which could be inhibited if clinicians felt compelled to follow a legal standard which fossilized a particular set of practices. A clearly argued exposition.

● Hirschfield EB (1993) Use of practice parameters as standards of care and in health care reform: a view from the American Medical Association. *J Qual Improvement.* **19**: 322–9.

Discussing practice parameters interchangeably with practice guidelines, the author argues that guidelines gain legal authority only as a consequence of their credibility with clinicians. Highly reliable practice parameters can thereby achieve a status approaching a mandatory standard of care. Guidelines can be used by a court to serve as reference points in assisting it to decide upon the applicable standard of care, rather than this standard of care being *constituted* by the guideline itself. He argues that because there is no agreed guideline taxonomy which could provide a court with an objective and independent view of a guideline's reliability or applicability, no guideline is likely to be credited with special legal authority *until* it has been shown in court to meet the common law requirement of wide professional acceptance and credibility.

● Hyams AL, Brandenburg BA, Lipsitz SR *et al.* (1995) Practice guidelines and malpractice litigation: a two-way street. *Ann Intrn Med.* **122**: 450–5.

This paper reports on one of the few empirical studies of the use to which clinical guidelines may be put in US malpractice suits. The authors sampled and reviewed the files of two professional liability insurance companies in the USA, including all the obstetric and anaesthetic claims. They also surveyed a 10% sample of attorneys across 50 states who specialized in medical malpractice. Of 259 insurance claims, only 17 (6.6%) involved a practice guideline which had had a 'pivotal role in the proof of negligence', 12 in an inculpatory capacity, and four in an exculpatory capacity. The authors comment that:

'... proponents of guidelines should be aware that the inculpatory use of guidelines in litigation may chill physicians' interest in developing more specific and prescriptive guidelines.'

Some 75% of responding attorneys were aware of clinical practice guidelines, 27% reporting their existence to have influenced a decision to settle a case and 26% reporting that guidelines had been influential in decisions not to pursue a case in the previous year. The authors therefore believe that guidelines could play an important role in pre-trial screening, helping to ensure that more meritorious cases are filed against doctors and brought to court, and that inappropriate cases which lack merit could be thrown out at an early stage of an action. Attorneys did not seem to think that guidelines influenced the need for medical experts in court, only 4.7% believing that they had decreased such a need, while 11.8% felt that guidelines had increased the need for medical experts. The majority of attorneys agreed that guidelines had made no difference.

• Kinney ED and Wilder MM (1989) Medical standard setting in the current malpractice environment: problems and possibilities. *Univ Cal at Davis Law Review*, **22**; 421–50.

The authors discuss US legal procedures by which practice guidelines may be introduced into courts as evidence of customary practice in cases of malpractice. They believe that clinical guidelines and protocols drawn up by professional associations provide a much better chance that defendant doctors will be held to a *consensual* standard of diagnosis and treatment, rather than an idiosyncratic standard of care put forward as customary by an expert witness but which may not be sufficiently tested by court proceedings. Liberal references to primary case law materials and secondary legal literature.

• Mehlman MJ (1990) Assuring the quality of medical care: the impact of outcome measurement and practice standards. *Law Med Health Care*. **18**: 368–84.

A comprehensive and accessible review of the role of medical standards and practice guidelines in the context of US health care. In Mehlman's view, the Maine 5-year Medical Demonstration Project is too one-sided in allowing *compliance* with guidelines to be cited as *exculpatory* evidence by defendant physicians, but *excluding* these guidelines from a role as *inculpatory* evidence for use by plaintiff patients. Such asymmetry may violate the requirements of due process and equal protection of the US Constitution. The paper's 117 annotated references are particularly valuable.

• Leahy RE (1989) Rational health policy and the legal standard of care: a call for judicial deference to medical practice guidelines. *Cal LR*. 77: 1483–528.

A rallying call for those who believe rationally developed guidelines should *determine* doctors' actions, the paper argues that practice guidelines should not only influence malpractice actions but could practically do so if courts were to take judicial notice of them *as constituting* the legal standard of care. This would replace the current situation in the USA in which a jury both decides the minimum required standard, and whether the standard has been met in the particular case before it. A procedure of judicial notice of guidelines would establish the standard of care for the jury whose job it would then be to decide, on the basis of the standard set out by the judge, whether the standard had been met by the particular facts of the case.

• National Health Lawyers Association (1995) Colloquium Report on Legal Issues Related to Clinical Practice Guidelines. National Health Lawyers Association, Washington DC.

This report summarizes the discussions of 26 participants in a colloquium convened by the US National Health Lawyers Association, an educational non-partisan organization of some 7000 health care lawyers working in hospitals, government and university settings, and in private practice. Convened in order 'to crystallize the tensions that exist between many people affected by practice guidelines', the main body of the report provides a comprehensive discussion of the legal issues thrown up by guideline proliferation. The report addresses such questions as: what legal authority (and liability) do groups creating, validating or disseminating guidelines carry? What role can guidelines play in establishing a legally recognized minimum standard of health care? How may conflicts, which arise when a doctor's duty towards a particular patient seems to be at odds with clinical guidelines issued by a Health Maintenance Organization predominantly for gate-keeping reasons, be resolved? Should the creation and validation of practice guidelines be regulated centrally? The Report also includes the following noteworthy papers sent as background briefings to discussants:

– Gosfield AG (1994) *Clinical practice guidelines and the law: applications and implications* (pp. 61–95).

A well-referenced survey of the historical, organizational and managerial origins of US clinical guidelines which concludes that their major role lies in health care rationing. It examines the legal implications of guidelines at different levels of health care delivery, the author recognizing that the adequacy of guideline development processes is central to their legal standing.

− Kapp MB (1990) *'Cookbook' medicine: a legal perspective* (pp. 139–46).

In setting standards of health care Kapp argues that clinical guidelines and practice parameters are not new departures; what *is* new is the degree to which guidelines make standards explicit whilst at the same time providing a mechanism for imposing them upon clinicians. Such standards will inevitably be used against doctors in malpractice cases, but the author believes it to be preferable:

'for enforceable legal standards of care to be drawn from the consensus work of voluntary, informed, competent entities with appropriate medical experience than from the *ad hoc*, retrospective expert witness contests that currently dominate legal decision-making about medical standards.'

In his view, the courts appreciate that guidelines offer only presumptive advice, 'to be followed or modified in light of the physician's experience and judgment'. Clinical guidelines are therefore unlikely to result in significant liability to their issuers or developers. The paper is clear and accessible but provides few references to case law.

− Kapp MB (1995) *The legal status of clinical practice parameters: an annotated bibliography* (pp. 147–51).

Short annotations on 19 medico-legal papers examining the significance of practice parameters and clinical guidelines. Only one paper considers the issues from a UK perspective − the rest concern North America.

● Noble A, Brennan T and Hyams A (1998) Snyder v American Association of Blood Banks: a re-examination of liability for medical practice guideline promulgators. *J Evaluation in Clinical Practice*. In press.

A very thorough review of the implications of a recent US case, *Snyder v American Association of Blood Banks* (1996). During an operation in 1984 William Snyder received an HIV infected blood transfusion supplied by Bergen Community Blood Center and subsequently developed AIDS. He contended that the AABB had been negligent in failing to recommend the screening of donors by way of surrogate testing prior to August 1984. The initial court had found for the plaintiff, but the AABB appealed on the grounds that it was a third party with no immediate responsibility for patient care and could not have had a duty of care towards Mr Snyder. The Supreme Court of New Jersey recognized that the AABB had no direct involvement in obtaining or processing the blood used for transfusions by its members. But it argued that by 1983 the AABB should have foreseen that blood transfusions were likely to transmit AIDS. Because of its leading position in setting minimum standards in a self-governing industry, and its role in accrediting member institutions, it had a duty of care to patients. The paper discusses the implications of trade association liability to third parties for negligent standard setting for which the authors can find no medical malpractice precedents in US case law.

• Schockemoehl G (1984) Admissibility of written standards as evidence of the standard of care in medical and hospital negligence actions in Virginia. *Univ Richmond LR.* **18**: 725–49.

Starting from the premise that the degree of skill and care a defendant doctor requires to possess in order to avoid being found negligent is the elusive one of being possessed of the skill of a reasonably prudent practitioner, the author, a practising lawyer, makes a plea for the courts in Virginia to allow accepted medical standards and accreditation rules to be sufficient in and of themselves to establish the applicable standard of care in alleged cases of malpractice without the need for additional expert testimony. The paper outlines a set of possible procedural steps by which such standards could be introduced into courts. The paper offers a clear and accessible argument which provides a good legal background to the issues.

• Smith GH (1993) A case study in progress: practice guidelines and the affirmative defense in Maine. *J Qual Improvement.* **19**: 355–62.

A lucid account of the historical development and policy rationale behind the Maine Medical Liability Demonstration Project in the USA. With a statutory basis, the project has created state-wide, legally validated clinical guidelines admissible in court. Under the legislation, guidelines or protocols developed by the Maine Medical Association and adopted by state Licensing and Registration Boards may be cited as an affirmative defence to a malpractice suit once a defendant doctor can show that he or she has followed such a guideline in the case before a court.

• Schyve PM (1993) Judges as gatekeepers: guidelines in court. *J Qual Improvement.* **19**: 283–90.

This paper consists of an interview with a Chief Judge of the Milwaukee County Circuit Court and a senior lawyer from the Judicial Policy Studies, Centre for Health Policy Research at George Washington University. The main topics covered include the creation of a desk reference book to assist US judges in deciding what constitutes admissible scientific or medical testimony in court. Since the US Supreme Court ruling in *Daubert v Merrell Dow Pharmaceuticals Inc* (1993), scientific principles, techniques or discoveries upon which expert testimony may be based need not have gained wide acceptance in their own field. It is now up to US trial judges to assess factors such as the underlying reasoning or methodology of expert testimony, whether a guideline is scientifically valid and can be applied to the facts at issue, or whether any theory or technique upon which it is based has been tested or subjected to peer review, and whether its margin of error is known. Only if expert scientific or medical testimonies pass these judicial screening tests can they be made admissible to a jury. The desk book discussed in this paper is designed to educate judges in the area of how to assess the validity of practice guidelines and expert testimony.

• Spernak SM, Budetti PP and Zweig F (1992) *Use of Language in Clinical Practice Guidelines.* Center for Health Policy Research, Agency for Health Care Policy and Research. Rockville, MD. Manuscript available from National Technical Information Service, Springfield, Virginia, VA 22161 USA.

A carefully worded resource written by two lawyers and a physician, providing invaluable advice to guideline authors on how to phrase guidelines with a minimum of ambiguity. Particular emphasis is given to the semantic and possible legal significance of certain vocabularies and sentence structures. It points out a variety of drafting hazards, and provides useful tips on how to say what is intended. Concise and timely advice by experienced operators in the guidelines field, with a strong focus on possible guideline uses within the arena of US medical negligence actions.

Index